STRUGGLING TO BE WELL

My life story and triumph over Schizophrenia

Keith Vander Wees

Copyright © 2022 Keith Vander Wees

All rights reserved

No part of this book may be reproduced, or stored in a retrieval system, or transmitted in any form or by any means, electronic, mechanical, photocopying, recording, or otherwise, without express written permission of the publisher.

Some names have been changed to protect privacy.

ISBN: 9798792158160

Cover design by: Keith Vander Wees
Library of Congress Control Number: 2018675309

*Dedicated to all those who have suffered
spiritually, mentally, and physically.*

CONTENTS

Title Page
Copyright
Dedication
Introduction
Prologue

Early Years	9
The Smokes on You	39
Let Me Out!	43
Let's not and say we did	52
Golf Anyone?	61
The Band Years	67
Toronto, Home Again	94
A complete mental breakdown	152
Timelines I'm not sure of - 1989 to 93	207
Release from hospital - 1993	220
Another Dream	234
More Healing Time – 2005 to 2007	237
Love you Dad	254

Epilogue	257
Acknowledgement	259
About The Author	261
Books By This Author	263

INTRODUCTION

For a large part of this book I rarely mention mental illness as I had no idea exactly what was wrong with my thinking until my breakdown and diagnoses at age 30. This book is my life story, including my many battles with the demons of mental illness as well as winning the little wars along the way. It is my sincere hope that this book may be of help, give insight to others who suffer with mental illness and bring hope to their families.

PROLOGUE

I was scared, walking through the greenhouses and foaming at the mouth. I looked at a power panel thinking it had flames billowing out of it. The plants were giving off an odd, deep smell and everything looked and felt very otherworldly dark and scary. When my Dad saw me, he thought he should take me to the hospital and I agreed to go. It was the hospital I was born in and had been admitted twice as a child with Croup, this time seeing a psychiatrist who asked a bunch of questions that I was too afraid to answer. I tried to leave the room to get away but Dad stood in my way at the door blocking me. As I tried to get by him he grabbed me by my long hair leaving him with a handful. I frantically broke away, the psychiatrist yelling "no, no, let him leave!" I went outside and started wandering around not knowing what to do, feeling like I was someone else, not the musician I had been for years, that all seemed so far away now. The general hospital called the police who arrived in minutes and took me to the psychiatric hospital but I didn't recognize the building, thinking I had gone to another dimension and was no longer in this world.

This first hospital admission was 1 out of 9, I was put on meds, in the hospital for several weeks and was released to my parents, staying at their home. This admission was the easy one.

STRUGGLING TO BE WELL

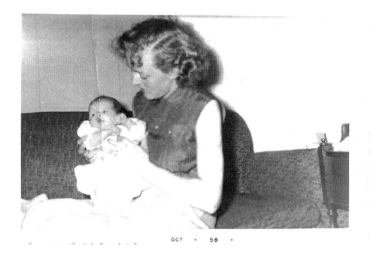

Mom and I - 1958

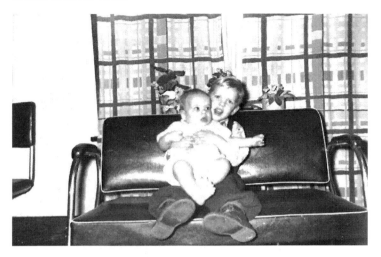

John and I - 1959

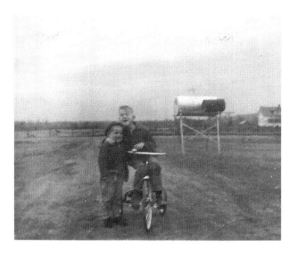

John and I - 1962

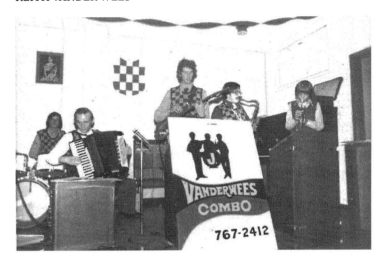

2nd Band I was with - 1973
Left to right -
Me, Howard, John, Jim, Ron (sitting in on trumpet)

STRUGGLING TO BE WELL

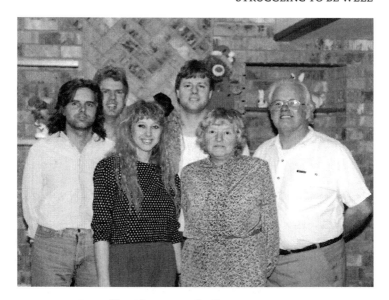

Family Photo - Christmas – 1989
Left To Right Back - Me, John, Rob, Dad
Left To Right Front - Bev, Mom

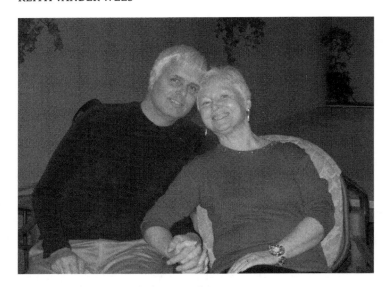

Elaine and I – 2009
At my parents' home in Thunder Bay

STRUGGLING TO BE WELL

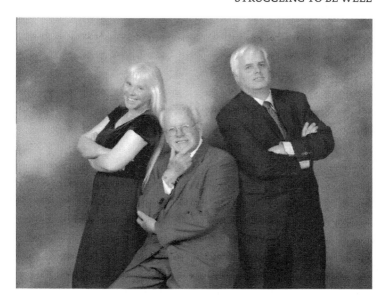

Charlie's Angels photo on a cruise – 2010
Bev, Dad, Me

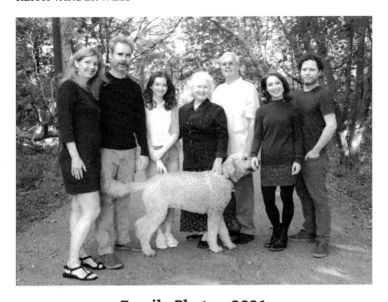

Family Photo – 2021
Left To Right - Jill, Steve, Evy, Elaine, Me, Laura, Sage,
and of course, Hoover the Dog

EARLY YEARS

I'd like to start with some family history, my journey is woven with early signs of mental illness. Also, our family history was integral to my spiritual growth and well-being.

My Dad came from a long line of greenhouse growers in Holland. He emigrated at the age of 22 along with his parents and seven of his siblings (Brother Jaap stayed behind) in the early 1950s to Oliver Township just outside of Port Arthur, Ontario. The family had bought 160 acres of property for $7,000 where they started a poultry farm selling eggs to stores. My Mom being born in Winnipeg, Canada but having both of her parents also from Holland, was 17 years old when moving to Port Arthur (which later amalgamated with the twin city of Fort William becoming Thunder Bay). After they married in 1954, Dad who was eager to learn the new language made a deal with Mom that if she would teach him English, he would teach her Dutch in return, as he spoke very little English when he first arrived. He had several jobs when he first came to Canada. One story was when he managed to get a job as an electrician at Canada Car (which in later years became Bombardier). It was a great job but with one minor detail, he wasn't an electrician. It didn't take them more than a few days to figure that out, and Dad took a job briefly working in the bush cutting timber.

My Mom also came from a large family having nine siblings, she being the eldest. Although she was a full time stay at home parent with two young boys (older brother John and I), my parents decided to take over a corner grocery store re-naming it Vans Grocery in 1957. In April 1960, my sister Bev was born and the lease on the store was running out at the end of the month. My Mom knew there was no way with three young kids that she could keep the business going with my Dad delivering Dutch products on the road during the day.

They packed everything up at the store and moved a house from the airport to a property in McIntyre, which was located in the country on a dirt road that was paved several years later. That house had no basement. We had a space heater and a stove, but there was no heat in the bedrooms. It was so cold in there that "Uncle" Hank (he was a very good friend of my parents and us kids always knew him as Uncle) and Dad got hay bales and put them all around the circumference of the house to keep the cold from coming in underneath. It was at this house that our last sibling brother Rob was born. Uncle Hank helped with the construction of a first humble greenhouse and that year Mom and Dad started growing bedding plants. Mom did the planting and watering etc., and left the heavy lifting to my Dad. All of this exemplifies just how hard-working my parents were and all four of us children have a strong work ethic which we learned from them. In the 1960s the transplanting was first done on tables, filling the packs by hand and shovel with soil that was stored underneath. Later as the business grew the pack filling was done by a hopper machine. The packs were then piled up on a pallet and shrink wrapped then brought from the soil building to the planting area by a bobcat machine. The ladies planted at a conveyer belt that had 3 seats on each side for them. Mom sat in on the planting for fun to shoot the breeze with the ladies at the greenhouse well into her 70s.

In the mid 1960s Dad decided to try his hand at being an independent egg delivery man, getting the eggs from his three brothers' chicken farm. For years, he would go door-to-door in town eventually creating many customers. Little did we know that years later forming relationships with all of these egg customers would play a large part in creating a whole new career path for my Dad. He had all his egg customer information in little books such as addresses and if they owed money. He also knew how many dozen they needed, and where at the house to leave the eggs if no one was at home. As kids, one or two of us at a time would go delivering with Dad on a Saturday. Sometimes when we were out delivering Dad would come back to the truck and tell me there was a lady asking about me in a house. I'd get reeled in and say, "really?" feeling like a rock star. He'd say, "she was asking who the fine young gentleman was sitting in the van." That's when I knew he was making that up. Sometimes it would be at the bank, but he always would fool me with that story. Even though it was a silly prank it always made me laugh in a groaning type of way. "Daaaad!" I'd say, like I wanted him to stop but I loved that he paid attention to me. As we got older, we would notice the telltale sign of a smile on one side of his face when he was about to pull the wool over our eyes.

There was a lady that would come outside to the van every week and ask "How mucha?" for the eggs. Dad would say 66 cents a dozen. She'd always say "Too mucha!" This happened every week until after about a month she again asked how much to which my Dad replied "40 cents a dozen." "I'll take 6 dozen!" she replied excitedly. "Sorry," Dad said, "Sold out!" and he moved on to the next house. There were always the people who having been used to bartering for things in their native countries, would try to get him to give them a better price for the eggs. Dad always took this in stride. He always had a great sense of humour and loved to get people laughing (either with him or at him). Once with Dad on the egg route we were parked at the last customer of the day's house in the driveway on top of a hill. Dad went in for a few minutes, but since the emergency hand brake hadn't been pressed the truck started to roll slowly down the hill toward the highway. John Brink, son of the house owner saw it from the picture window, came running out, jumped in the truck and stopped the vehicle before it got near the highway. He made sure I was o.k. and my Dad got in and drove us home. Of course, it didn't dawn on me (being about five years old) that I was in any danger at all, so, when we were at that house a week later my Dad went in once again and I took off the emergency brake myself. It was amazing I thought, as the van rolled down the hill like some kind of ride that I got going myself. Again, John Brink came running out and stopped the van, this time being very angry with me. That time I was in a lot of trouble with my Dad.

My Dad also sold Dutch products along with the eggs at one point. There were lovely, tasty chocolate letters, that at four years old I enjoyed eating when he was out of the truck. The letters just started to disappear, and it didn't take long for him to catch on who was eating the profits.

Certain things happened in our family to Dad that could only happen to a cartoon character. A classic Dad story which we love to tell as a family is him on his way to Holland with Keith, one of his brothers to visit another brother Jaap and his wife Celia. Dad and Keith both had been drinking on the plane when Dad went to the washroom. As he was just finishing up in there, he coughed, his false teeth falling into the toilet and getting flushed in with the blue water. Dad tried to retrieve them but to no avail, ending up with a blue arm for the rest of the flight. Imagine him toothless, trying to explain to his brother when he got back to his seat, where his teeth went and how he got the blue arm.

When they arrived at Jaap and Celia's apartment Celia asked Dad what he'd like to eat. Dad, toothless, replied "I think I'll have the thoup." Not liking being without teeth, Dad had a pair made in Holland that were like big chompers which he aptly called Horse Teeth. Once he got back to Canada, he had another pair of teeth made and was a lot happier with those.

Another time, Dad got up from his afternoon nap and came into the greenhouse walking very gingerly and looking confused. He told Mom he felt unwell, had blurry vision and a headache. Mom said, "you better go lay down for a while, take it easy, and when you get up again put your own glasses on." Of course, my Dad wasn't too impressed but it is obvious that my Mom has a very creative sense of humour that sneaks up on you.

Another great Dad story is he had just bought a brand-new full length leather coat and was very proud of it. A few days after buying it he got in his car and threw it in the back seat not realizing that 3/4 of it was hanging out between the door when he closed it. As he was driving, the coat got tangled up in the back wheel. Eventually he saw his lovely coat, his lovely new coat all ripped to shreds. Of course, this story along with others became family favourites to repeat and he'd always laugh along in the retelling. Dad always was kind and thoughtful and every morning since he was up first, he would bring Mom a cup of coffee in bed letting her wake up slowly. Mom just loved this.

My older brother John was born in 1955, me in 1958, sister Bev in 1960 and youngest sibling Rob was born in 1962. Our family farm had a dog, two Siamese cats, ducks, geese, chickens, rabbits and pigs as well as a large bountiful garden. Unfortunately, we lost a lot of our dogs to getting hit by cars. Another little drawback of country living for us was Kurt, our middle aged and completely bald neighbor having four or five cows that would often break down a flimsy dividing fence between our properties and come into our garden for a feast. It seemed very often during the milder seasons that Dad, frustrated, was on the phone telling

Kurt that the cows were back. Kurt would promptly come over with his whip and crack it in the air loudly to scare the cows back to his yard. He was constantly fixing that fence but Dad, even with this minor aggravation still would often have him over for a drink. One afternoon after several drinks Kurt rode his tractor to the main highway and was trying to Lasso cars that were passing by at a high rate of speed. He was very lucky he didn't rope one.

Back in those days the twin cities of Port Arthur and Fort William were only a few miles apart and each had their own mayor and city council. At that time both cities had many industries for high paying jobs. Grain elevators and a thriving pulp and paper industry kept many people employed, along with Canada Car. The grain elevators and pulp and paper industries have disappeared and in recent years the trains and buses have stopped coming into the city as well. Now, the only way in or out of Thunder Bay is by car, plane or boat, leaving the port city of Thunder Bay seeming even more isolated. It is a beautiful scenic area with the large 'Sleeping Giant' rock formation in the harbour visible from many vantage points and Kakabeka Falls and Ouimet Canyon being only a few examples of many of nature's wonders in the area. The city is remote with the nearest large city Winnipeg, Manitoba, 500 miles to the West. Toronto, Ontario, is 1000 miles to the southeast with miles and miles of trees in between. Duluth, Minnesota, a city with a slightly smaller population than Thunder Bay is 200 miles to the south and it's only about a 40-minute drive to the U.S border.

One day when I was about three, I was outside in the yard playing service station attendant. Later that day Mom wanted to go to the store, so she packed up all four kids and we all got in the car. We got about 100 feet down the road toward the store and the car died. Mom couldn't figure out what was going on with the car, so I said, "I know we have gas, I just filled it up" She replied, "Filled it up? with what?" I said, "With the hose!" feeling very proud. At first Mom thought Oh no, but then kind of laughed. When my Dad got home, he and Uncle Hank had to take the gas tank off and dry everything out. There were times I was tethered to the clothesline for my own safety to keep me from getting into mischief all the time or from getting hit by a car.

There was a night when I was about 4 that our parents were across the street visiting the neighbours in the wee hours. An aunt of ours who was babysitting us was fast asleep on the couch. I had been sleeping till then but now was restless. With the trust and naive bravery of a child I climbed out the window in my pjs and bare feet and walked across our lawn which had an early morning frost layer. I was on a mission, crossing a country road which had no traffic that time in the morning. I knocked on the neighbour's door and when someone answered they didn't see me for a second until they looked down, then shouted, "Keith!!" Dad and Mom came to the door and brought me home. Dad wrapped me up in his long coat to keep me warm. I don't know what was warmer, the coat or my heart from feeling loved and protected.

Many mornings at age 4, I would open the kitchen cupboard underneath the sink and drag out all the pots and pans I could handle. I would then bring them into the living room, and with forks and table knives, play my heart out to the test pattern music on the T.V. I made quite a racket, even having a little top from a pot as a cymbal. It was my first experience with drumming of any kind, and I seemed to have natural rhythm. After a year or so of pots and pans I gave up drumming for several years.

I was always an inquisitive child, loving to take things apart, look at them and explore and learn about how they worked. The only problem was I could never remember how to put any of them back together. We ended up having a lot of broken things including my poor Dads beautiful pump organ. I started taking that apart piece by piece until finally my Dad had enough and threw it in the backyard saying, "Go to it", but I lost interest since it was no longer a challenge anymore and I probably enjoyed the ambience of the house more for deconstruction than the great outdoors. It was about this age that I would start spending hours a day lying down in my room when no one was around rocking only my head side to side to the beat of music playing to try to calm some of the anxiety I was feeling. I would continue to do this over the years even into my early 30s until I recovered from mental illness. I've always been very embarrassed about this, never telling anyone before, but some may have been aware of it hearing a rhythmic squeaking noise coming from the bed springs.

I used to play Keith the Martian at about 6 years old, Bev was 4. I would tell her that Keith the Martian was coming and then I'd be mean to her. She'd always plead with me "But I don't want Keith the Martian to come out!" Thank goodness I got out of doing that quickly. At a young age I didn't seem to have a lot of empathy for others. I was self-absorbed. At around the same age, I'd break a toy or something on purpose and tell my parents that Rob (who was just 2 years old) had actually done it, just to get him into trouble until he got old enough and could explain for himself what really happened. I was then on the receiving end of a spanking for lying. I remember getting some sick pleasure when he would get into trouble and get a spanking. I do believe my mental challanges started even at this early age. I've always felt so bad with regret about terrorizing both Bev and Rob, but I did eventually become a better person having more empathy for others.

Around the time I started to ride a bike I got in the habit of playing little games in my mind. As I'd be riding toward home, I'd often count the telephone poles thinking that if the number I chose in my head was exactly the number of poles when I reached our yard, I'd live to see another day. Even though I was always hopeful that the count would be correct, starting at a very young age I was always afraid of dying and more than likely had O.C.D. This is another possible early sign that something was not right with my mental well being. Even to this day, often at night I count the second hand ticking from an analog clock in the living room and count how many seconds till our digital clock in the bedroom number changes. If I guess right with how many seconds till the clock changes it makes me feel more at ease like I am on the right life path, and that I have made a divine connection with God who lead me to guess right. Unfortunately, I struggle with my faith and need constant reasurrace that God is with me.

One winter afternoon on a Saturday, when I was about 8 years old, I was helping Dad on the egg route, which I always enjoyed. Dad was backing out of a yard and missed the driveway, putting the truck part way in a deep ditch on an angle. Dad tried a couple of times to keep backing out, but if he had kept going the truck would have tipped right over. It was on such a drastic angle, I had to crawl out of my door to pull myself out of the van. Dad went into the house and called for a tow truck from the local service station he used quite often. Sam, the tow truck guy that came out to help us, probably in his 60s at the time, was very nervous about trying to pull us out. He told my Dad if something happened, he wasn't responsible. My Dad told him not to worry about it, just go ahead and pull the van out. Sam hooked a chain up to the back of the van. After about three or four very careful tries, the tow truck slowly pulled us out without tipping us over. I didn't know then that later at age 16 I would work at that service station for several months doing full service like pumping gas, checking oil and cleaning windshields. This was typical service back then and working there was a great way for me to start interacting with people more.

I developed a lifetime fear of deep water after going to swimming classes at the YMCA. I always enjoyed the showers there which were so hot and steamy, feeling so good. The shower was a release for me for some of the anxiety I was always feeling. At home we only had a bathtub at first, so these were my first showers ever. The classes were taking place on the weekends, starting off for several weeks in the shallow end. I did look forward to them at first. One week we started to work on laying on our back and just floating, which I was at first very tentative about but was able to do. Shortly after that day they had me jump in the deep end. I panicked, yelling for help and splashing anxiously, going under a few times. They had to pull me out of the water. I never went back and still don't swim, so afraid, even though several people have tried to teach me. Now, I will go into water but not where it's any deeper than my waist.

Over the years my Mom has mentioned that she figured she was quite immature at the time she was having us kids, but we always felt that we were loved, and I think that's the most important thing. No matter what, there was a lot of love in our house even though like normal siblings we didn't always get along. If we were playing outside at mealtimes, Mom would yell out the doorway for us to come home. We might have been 2 or 3 country houses away, but we could hear her calling and would race home to a hearty home cooked meal.

My eldest brother John was always very protective and straightened out several kids in school that were picking on me.

I've always felt very close to John. The first time I was admitted to the psychiatric hospital he came to see me and was crying. It hurt my heart, but I really saw how much he cared about my struggles with mental health. My sister Bev was always very protective of Rob, the youngest in the family. When a boy would pick on him, Bev, who is by nature very kind and gentle, would hit them over the head with her lunch pail. Several times a particular family would be calling that Bev had beat up their boy.

Our Grandfather on Mom's side had gifted us with a shuffleboard (called Sjoelbak in Holland), we played often and became very good at it. The game consisted of sliding the flat, rounded wooden stones on a board through small slots at the other end barely big enough to pass the stone through. We'd shoot them so hard that sometimes they would jump out the back of the board, hitting the patio door window. I think Rob and I still disagree who ended up as the all-time champ.

Younger brother Rob and I were very

competitive, playing hockey outside in boots instead of skates, just the 2 of us, one in net, and one shooting. With the long winter months and tons of snow we also made snow forts and threw snowballs at passing cars, ducking down after the impact. The drivers were none too pleased with this activity. They would catch us, but we took the heat and kind of laughed it off when they would drive off (that is until my Mom and Dad found out and that was the end of that game). Gleefully riding our bikes in winter into the snow filled ditch and flying off the bike into the white blanket was also a favourite pastime. We'd have great fun and laughed a lot.

Spaghetti and Soup

Bev and I had times in our lives that we would be at odds with each other. At mealtimes when we were kids, I would make a point during an argument and rub it in, making the point over and over till she'd had more than enough. Boom! I'd have either a plate of spaghetti in my lap or a bowl of soup over my head depending upon what was on the menu that day.

I would just sit there briefly afterwards shocked but cleaned the mess up before my parents saw it. I should've known it was coming. It happened so many times (until I got smart and kept my big mouth shut).

Bev has quite a few lifelong friends. When they were very young, she and one friend with whom she is still close, loved animals so much they called themselves the "Animal Queens." They would spend many a day playing in the forest singing "We love animals 1-2-3" (a sweet song they made up) and were very creative making up their own words like "Trunto," "Danekin" and "Dunabug." Bev continues to be very creative writing daily journal entries.

Many fun filled but hard-working summers were spent at my Grandparents farm. I have an uncle (Ed) that's only two years older than me, so we were childhood friends. I would go over there for a few weeks at a time during the summer, but it wasn't all fun and games. We had to work as we got older which I found challenging but really didn't mind at all. We'd get up in the morning at a reasonable hour and would help grandpa in the fields or packing produce in the dugout under the house (there was no basement). It wasn't very hard work, mostly picking vegetables in the fields, or weeding. The reward was after supper we would get to go tubing at the creek or whatever else we wanted to do. Tubing down the small rapids of the shallow, waist-deep creek was a great joy in that time of my life. The only downside was when we got to the pool of water at the end we'd have to get out before the bloodsuckers attached themselves. If there were any on us, a dash of salt would remove them.

When we were younger, before we had to work, in the afternoon Grandma would make cold tea in a mason jar for us to bring to Grandpa, who was working in the hot sun in the fields. He was always so grateful, taking huge swigs of the wet, refreshing tea. Ed and I had no shortage of games to play. On the farm, there were lots of little nooks and crannies to play in. We were great friends during those years with Ed teaching me all the berries and nuts on the property that were safe to eat and even how to spot wild chamomile to make tea. On Sundays we would wake up to the smell of bacon cooking and head to the Christian Reformed Church for about 10 am. The minister was always very entertaining in his sermon, with his hands flailing around like he was going to fly off the pulpit. It was like I wanted to look away, but my eyes kept drifting back to watching him. With Grandpa being very religious we couldn't work at all on Sunday, not even fix a bike tire. Sunday evenings we had to endure the Dutch language service at the Church. The peppermints and other candies Grandma would give us for both services would help immensely and make things more interesting. Thankfully, the Dutch service was only about an hour. We hardly understood a word as we only spoke English at home.

When I was between the ages of 10 and 12, Mom would take me to a couple of the Bingo Halls that would let underage kids play. We'd always get there so early that the person responsible for opening up the hall would arrive after us. I always thought that was funny. Bingo was serious business to these ladies, and they all brought their favourite little lucky charms which they would line up on the table like little soldiers in front of their cards. One Bingo night was always held at a Roman Catholic Church in the basement that was located way out on a lonely country road. There were always a couple friendly games of cards at our table with several of the ladies before the Bingo proceedings. The thick cigarette smoke would fill the hall packed with about a hundred ladies and me, so bad that my eyes would be burning and the only way I could get relief was to put my head under the table. Mom would nervously watch my cards and hers, shouting "Bingo!!!" even before I had a chance to realize that I had won. I have always thought of myself as lucky, so when I would win a jackpot, Mom would share the winnings with all of the family. This was rightly so, as she paid for the Bingo cards.

When I was 12 years old, we went to a country fair. We were walking around quite a bit and somebody from a newspaper stopped us and asked if they could take a picture of me for the local newspaper. My parents and I thought that was great and it ended up in the paper several days later. In the photo I was holding a goose and the caption said "Best in class" sadly it was the goose that was best in class not me. I was terrible at school. I'd always drift off as soon as the teacher started talking as I could just not focus. By the time I got to Grade 8, I was lost. I always had music rolling around in my head and would tap out a beat with pencils or whatever would serve as drumsticks. A teacher actually wrote on one of my report cards "If Keith spent as much time on his studies as he does drumming on his desk..." They kept advancing me even though I hadn't done the work and by Grade 9 I was functioning at a Grade 5 math level as well as many of the other subjects. I was very well spoken at a young age. My reading and spelling levels were also very good, so they probably kept moving me on for those reasons. Even though I have very little education I've never let that hold me back and I've never had feelings of being hard done by.

My Dad also worked so hard. In the early 1970's, he went into politics. He was on the school board initially and then became a city councillor, which led to a political career that totalled more than 30 years. He didn't get in right away to the school board. It took him several tries. He even tried his hand at running for Mayor and as a member of Provincial Parliament. We were always so proud of him and his accomplishments. In Thunder Bay, Dad became very well known for his flowing silver locks and extremely positive and approachable personality. You always knew where you stood with Dad, and he wasn't afraid to take a stand on something that was right but maybe controversial. Everywhere he went, pretty much everyone knew him, which says a lot since the city population was over 100,000 people. There is a really great video on YouTube with the former mayor of Thunder Bay, Walter Assef, having a meeting with City Council. In this meeting as with many other Council meetings, Walter is off the rails and is chastising all kinds of people and belittling them. He threatens my Dad that he's going to whip him and my Dad says, "I wish you would!" I was so proud of Dad's quick response and still crack up every time I see it. Unbelievably, this video was a typical City Council meeting in the early 1980s. If you search on YouTube for Walter Assef you should be able to find it.

Like a lot of other kids, I was severely bullied in school, and beaten up almost daily. Some of the kids would call me "Teeth" instead of Keith because of the buck teeth I acquired from sucking my thumb for the first 8 years of my life. I was always feeling on edge and out of control, even at this young age and sucking my thumb and the rocking helped soothe that. They also called me Vander Chicken in relation to my uncle's egg farm. There were many times in my childhood that I just told my Mom I was too sick to go to school, which wasn't the truth. It was just that I didn't want to get beaten up again.

In my youth, I was often drumming away with my fingers on the back of an acoustic guitar that John owned. At one point, John mentioned to Mom and Dad how good he thought I sounded, and that year for my birthday I was delighted to receive a snare drum with a beautiful mother of pearl shell. Soon after, I bought my first drum set for 75 dollars, carefully sanded them down and repainted them, reselling them for 150 so I could buy a better set.

By grade 6, a few kids in my school and I formed a rock band called 'Sunburst' which all of a sudden made me one of the cool kids and then I wasn't bullied at all anymore. We played the local Community Centres and even the psychiatric hospital, where I ended up as a patient years later. Around this time, I had a little girlfriend, (my first crush) although in our age group we called it going around with someone. It was all very innocent; I think I kissed her one time with closed lips. She used to come to the dances at various Community Centres our band would play at. A couple of times during the show, the lead singer would take over the drums and I'd get to slow dance with her. I think my illness was affecting me already as I broke up with her numerous times not being able to handle the emotions I was feeling. I was paranoid, always thinking she was going to break up with me, so I'd do it first, so afraid of being rejected. I remember once telling her I had to break up with her because I was hooked on Hashish but at that point, I had not even tried drugs. I wasn't playing some game with her feelings; I was really struggling mentally and living in a constant state of fear and confusion. She was such a sweet girl; she deserved much better than being treated in that way.

Also In Grade 6, one day at school, somebody brought a beer from home, and we all went hiding down the hill by the school and shared it, thinking that it was the greatest thing. Funny thing was I didn't even like the taste of beer yet. One of the kids got the idea that we could bring more beers from home, so I got myself together the next morning took about 4 beers from Dad's case and put on my winter jacket. With an opener and the beer in my jacket pockets, I started up the stairs to catch the bus for school. I was clink-clinking up the stairs when my Mom stopped me at the top and asked me where I was going with my winter jacket on. I said nervously, "I think it might rain outside." What didn't work with that story was that it was a beautiful sunny summer day, not a cloud in the sky. She said, "Let me see in your pockets." I didn't really want to show her but of course I let her look in my pockets and the jig was up; I was caught with the beer. She wasn't very happy and said, "Wait till Dad gets home." All day at school, I dreaded about going home to face Dad. Mom told him what happened, but he seemed to be more amused than anything to my great relief. Dad, having several brothers himself, knew what kind of mischief young boys could get into. I never did it again.

THE SMOKES ON YOU

Of course, Uncle Ed and I did get into a little bit of trouble over the years as well. When I was about 14 years old, Ed was staying over at our place during the summer. We bought a can of Old Chum tobacco at the corner store, saying it was for my Mother. Deciding that it was too dangerous to bring it home, after we had smoked some, we thought we would hide it in the bush under a little piece of moss so we could find it again. We got home, were going to bed later that evening and my Mom said to me "Good night Old Chum!" A chill ran up my spine, I knew we were caught! Somebody must've seen us go into the bush, or the store clerk had given us up. We went back the next day to look for our stash but of course the can was gone.

Over the years our parents took in foster children who stayed with us when we were growing up. We had a teenage boy that took off from our home and was picked up by the police. We also had a heavy-set boy staying with us who would baby sit us and sit on us until we said "Uncle." He would also carry me outside at night and threaten to throw me in the pig pen. Mom and Dad didn't know about this until I told them years later when I was in my twenties. Some of these kids stayed in contact with my parents after they left our home. For a couple years we had two little First Nations sisters aged 4 and 9 living with us. Mom and Dad used to treat them like their own, buying them the same amount of Christmas presents and Dad bouncing them on his knee while he sang Dutch children's songs to them. After their own father recovered, the girls went back to live with him. We have kept in touch with them all these years as they're an important part of our family, even attending Mom's 80th birthday party.

One summer at around age 14, I went over to a friend's place to hang out. My friend, his younger brother, and myself ended up going to the barn where we went upstairs into the hayloft. There was an old go kart in the corner, and my friend got the idea that we should sniff the gas and see what happens. I was game for it and didn't see any immediate danger. We took turns sticking our noses and mouths in the gas tank, breathing in heavily, nothing happened for a while, so we kept doing it until sounds started reverberating and echoing in the hayloft. Suddenly somebody yelled "Echo, Echo, Stop!" I was right out of it and I saw a huge arrow come down in front of me and I melted down into and through the floor. I wasn't in the hayloft anymore, but in some other room which felt like a basement. There was a huge fleshy square thing that had people's faces in it, turning over and over making sounds like *boop-be-boop ... boop-be-boop*, over and over. It was madness and was so real, like reality times ten. I'd never had a feeling like that before. I was totally not in control, and it seemed like I was part of a movie that I was also watching. A voice said, "There's no such thing as the world, there is no such thing as your parents." I was in that state completely gone from this world for a few minutes it seemed, then coming out of it sitting on my butt with my legs crossed and a very loud ringing in my ears. I couldn't move and felt helpless, that I had lost my mind. After a bit, I moved again and asked my friend what happened, what he saw. He told me that he had also gone somewhere else but he had gone to a wheat field, and he was shredded by some kind of musical harp. My little bit of madness stayed with me for a lot of years and whenever I thought of that room I was in, it would start to feel that I was going back, and it would scare the crap out of me. I still can't think about it without being afraid. I wonder now if this gas sniffing experiment caused brain damage and triggered my mental illness later. I've never asked a doctor about it and that was the only time I ever sniffed gas or anything else.

LET ME OUT!

As a 14 year old, I used to hitchhike quite a bit into town and back, about 10 miles each way. One day, on the way back home, I got a ride with a fellow in a truck with a topper on it. I got in and immediately felt uncomfortable, there was something about him that creeped me out, and there was a smell in the truck I didn't like at all. He barely spoke and when we got to the place where I was going to get dropped off by the corner store, he sped up. "It's right here!" I shouted. "It's right here!", but he kept going faster and faster. I tried to open the door but for some reason it wouldn't open. I don't remember if it didn't have door handles or if the door just wouldn't open. Almost paralyzed with fear, I started to open the window to jump out, but then he slowed down and stopped. Just as I was getting out, he asked if I would take five dollars to give him a blow job. I told him to get lost or something like that and very, very nervously got out of the vehicle. I didn't tell my parents all about it till several days later, I was pretty embarrassed about the whole thing.

When I was 15, I volunteered in the Militia band with my brother John though he was paid because he was of age. The conductor told me about a 6-week Army Cadet course in Vernon B.C that was being offered. There was a Band Company that I could join while there, which I did when I arrived at the camp in mid-June. On the site there were many buildings which housed about 500 other cadets from all over Canada. I quickly made friends with 2 guys, Rick and Larry. During rifle training I was very nervous because even though I was in the Militia Band I'd never fired a rifle. On this day, we were learning about and going to be firing a very powerful FN rifle. Most of the day was spent learning safety, taking it apart and then reassembly. I didn't remember any of it and knew that most of the kids already had some experience with firearms.

Once we got to the field I was petrified

and shaking, so nervous. Everyone was dressed in green army fatigues except me, they had me in white (Being a novice, so everyone could keep an eye on me). I took my rifle, remembering to press it into in the meat of my shoulder, and aimed it at my target. I was way off, quite possibly hitting the target beside mine. Of course with some bad luck, the next bullet got jammed in my rifle (very dangerous). The Sergeant in charge fixed that for me and I was relieved that I was done for that part of the training. The rest of the day was spent in the wild learning to make a lean-to and participating in war games in teams. I made it through five weeks of training out of six which also included a 4-day trip in a Hercules Aircraft to Whitehorse for about 100 of us. It was quite cool in The Yukon at night even though it was the end of July and the sun never went down, it just skipped along the horizon. During our stay we did a little march through concert at a mall there, and later at night saw an amazing display of the northern lights, which we watched in awe. Once we got back to B.C, we were all glad to be back at camp.

One afternoon, one of my new friends got the idea that about six of us should pool our money together and buy some booze. I was already smoking at that time with a forged note from home that said I was fine to smoke while at the camp. We drew straws, and Rick and I were the chosen ones. The two of us cautiously walked up the highway to downtown hoping no one would see us and waited outside the liquor store for a possible booze buyer (someone old enough to buy it) for our night of fun. After asking several people with no success, one guy coming out said he would buy it for us. We handed him the cash which included about five dollars in loose change. He came out, we had our booze, and headed back to camp as fast as we could sweltering in the Okanogan heat with our army fatigues on.

That night the six of us were having a great time getting hammered on hard stuff when one of the kids passed out, bringing even more attention to us. The Sergeant brought us into his quarters where the kid was passed out in a chair and asked, "Did you do this?" We came clean and admitted that we did, dreading the possible repercussions. The next day we went before the camp commander (a Lieutenant Colonel) and we were all going to be RTU'd (returned to unit) except one kid who cried and apologised profusely. The rest of us got sent home and didn't get paid since we were one week short of completing the six-week course.

I was put on a plane in Kelowna to make the flight to Vancouver airport and I had about an hour to make my connection back to Thunder Bay through Winnipeg. It was a long line up and for some reason the person at the check in counter kept moving me to the back of the line and by the time I got to the gate, I sadly watched my plane go up without me. By this time there were no more flights to Thunder Bay, so I called my parents to tell them I missed my flight. I got them out of bed at midnight, It was 9 pm in Vancouver, and they were not happy that I was being sent home for drinking. A few hours later, I seem to remember that the whole airport was closed except for

Security. I had a nice chat with one of the Security staff, told him my RTU story, and he let me sleep on a row of chairs. I woke up early in the morning, a little stiff from my bed of chairs to hear the airport hustle and bustle. I found a note and cash beside me. The note read: "Here's two bucks for smokes and coffee. I know what it's like, I was once in the army, too."

Our Militia band played at the local semi pro hockey games for the Thunder Bay Twins and performed for the Queen of England when she came to town. For the Queen's performance, I was the bass drummer at an outdoor park and was instructed to wait till someone yelled "By the left", and I had to hit one quick boom. They then would say "Quick March" and the approximately 500 Military would march off. Someone yelled something and I thought it was my cue. I excitedly did the boom (too soon) which had the Military and crowd all looking at me like, what was that?. I was sweating until finally he yelled "By the left!", I hit it again, heard "Quick March!", and we all started moving. I was just relieved to get the heck out of there.

I didn't think very logically as a kid and often would do strange things. An example of this was when our class had a trip planned to go to Centennial Park during the school year. The trip included enjoying the park and going for a little swim. Our teacher said that only those that could swim would be allowed in the water to which I lied and said I could swim. In the park there were some raised rocks near the water that some of the kids were sitting on in-between swims. I still had all my clothes on, and someone dared me to jump in which I did and landed in the water with a big belly flop. I had no idea the water was so deep; I couldn't touch bottom, and I immediately panicked calling out for help. A few of the kids jumped in and pulled me out of the water. I was exhausted but more embarrassed than anything else. I found out later that when the teacher realised I was struggling in the water she called out to the other kids for someone to jump in, one saying, "You go get him" and another saying "No, you go get him." Afterwards the teacher was very upset with me, and the school had to call my parents and tell them what happened. Also, I got the idea at one point when I was in Grade 9 that I would be better off on my own and I went to a friend's house after school to stay the night and planned to look for a job in the morning. I had been having a wide variety of emotions and thoughts of not being good enough to have the parents I did and thought that both they and I would be better off if I was on my own. I didn't call my parents to tell them where I was so they were incredibly worried. The next day I went to the pool hall, was hanging out there and who showed up but my brother John. He told me that Dad was in the car, was in tears, and they were both very worried. John pleaded with me to come home. I felt terrible and got in the car with them.

In my youth I started a little greeting card business that I found advertised in a comic book. I would drive my bike around neighbourhoods selling the cards. It was a successful little venture and I made enough points to buy a lovely transitor radio. Later on in my teens I tried my hand at several other jobs, pumping gas, working in a record store, selling shoes, as a gopher in the restaurant in Eaton's, and working for my Uncle Hank at The Current River Bakery in Thunder Bay. I had bad nightmares of falling into and being caught in Uncle Hank's big bread mixers, and a recurring dream of being chased by dinosaurs. In that dream, I'd hear the thump, thump, thump of the footsteps chasing after me which consumed me in fear. I had that dream for several years until one night I woke up in the middle of the dream and realized that the thumping sound I was hearing was my own heart beating so hard from being scared. After that realization that dream disappeared.

LET'S NOT AND SAY WE DID

I only went as far as part of Grade 10 in school. In Grade 9 I was always hanging around with a group of kids that were known to get into a lot of trouble. The school did call my parents at one point to have a meeting about my choice of friends. Some of those kids were into break and enters, stealing cars and a lot of drugs. Since we lived in the country, I was able to avoid going along with any of their bad choices except for smoking a little marijuana sometimes at school. One day, just after school ended, one of my so-called friends wanted to go and steal a car and asked me if I wanted to come along with a group of them. I declined. That night they went out, stole the car and had over a pound of marijuana with them. They got caught, were charged with auto theft, possession and trafficking of marijuana and were in big trouble. One of them ended up in prison because he had a criminal past and had been in front of a judge many times prior to that. He owed money for the drugs that were confiscated by police and when he got out of prison, the drug dealers somehow got him to go into the pool hall, calling his parole officer who came down and saw for himself that he had violated his parole by being there. He was sent back to prison. One of the other kids ended up getting caught for all the break and enters. I am thankful and never regretted not going with those guys doing any of their break-ins or stealing things.

Later that year a friend of mine had an idea to light a little fire in the washroom of the school which I went along with. We weren't trying to light a big fire or hurt anyone, we just wanted to see what would happen if we lit a toilet paper roll on fire. It was a stupid idea. We didn't realize the roll would smoke so much, and the alarms went off while we were still in the washroom. We panicked, running out into the hall, with the whole school emptying out on to the sidewalk.

It was then too late when the seriousness of what we did really hit me. We were brought before the Vice Principal the next day, having been seen coming out of the washroom by someone. He was very angry with us, rightly so, and said that if we went to see a psychiatrist the school wouldn't call the police or bring in the Fire Marshal. We agreed to this. I saw a psychiatrist who just asked me a few questions, and said he knew that I really didn't intend to do any harm, it was just a stupid prank going too far. He said, "I'll tell your parents you're not all fucked up." I was never so happy to hear somebody swear that way and extremely relived. Around this time, I was often in the pool hall during school hours. One day someone came up to me and said, "Did you hear about Jeff?" I said "No, what?" he told me Jeff, my best friend, had committed suicide by shooting himself. I was shocked and devastated but realised knowing him well, that he was really messed up. Jeff was into Satan worshiping, Satanic records, had a goat's head etc., and his girlfriend had just broken up with him. Everything was just too much for him. Most of my friends and I were smoking quite a bit of marijuana around this time which only made my paranoia worse. I don't think I ever liked smoking it, I was stupidly going along with the rest of my friends. One thing I never did was acid or any other hallucinogenic drugs which my friends did a lot of. I think that if I had it might have been the end of what little sanity I had left.

That summer, I went downtown on a weekend and met up with a friend. He suggested we buy a bottle of rum, and it was decided that I was the one going in the liquor store for it. I was really surprised when I walked up to the counter put the bottle and the money down, and they didn't stop me from buying it being only 16 years old. I felt like I had just robbed a bank. We drank most of it and my friend decided to leave. I was totally smashed and started wandering around downtown, going into a movie theatre to see Blazing Saddles. I could barely focus on the screen, so I left the theatre taking a bus across town to the Fort William area. I threw up and passed out in an alleyway next to a jewellery store where the owner came out and asked if I was okay. I asked them to call a taxi which arrived, I got in and the driver asked to see the money before leaving to take me home. I told him I'd pay him when we got there, but he said no way and told me to get out as he wasn't going to take me anywhere. I opened my door and fell out of the car saying to him "You don't even care if I die do you?" He said, "No I don't!" and left. Feeling dejected, I took the bus back to Port Arthur across town and staggered into 'Crazy Mike's Music' store that my friend's father owned. They called my parents and my Mom picked me up. When I got home, I told my parents that I was in the washroom at the movie theatre and two guys forced me to drink the alcohol. They somehow believed that story until many years later I told them the truth. That evening I had a gig with my brother's band playing drums at a special engagement and I could barely play from the hangover I had; I learned a lesson, if only for a few days.

When I was about 16, I quit school and got a job at Shaws Bakery. The new guy was always the pan man, taking the hot pans off the conveyor belt. The gloves they provided were inadequate, were old and had holes in them so I was feeling the hot pans. During my first day on the job, I was trying to show them that I could be a hard worker. The break bell went off, but I took my break after diligently cleaning up with a broom for five minutes. By the time I got back five minutes later than everyone else from break, the pans were all backed up, jammed all along the huge conveyer. The supervisor was quickly pulling the backlogged pans apart yanking them off the line. I had no idea the whole system was timed; he was furious with me. Everything on the line was timed including the ovens which held about a hundred pans with four loaves in each of them, so any little hiccup was a big deal. Eventually I started to have some back issues from the heavy lifting and was put on lighter and lighter work. Finally, after continually complaining about my back to the supervisor, I was told at the end of a workday that I would have to do a double shift that day and stay another 8 hours. I refused. I told him that my Dad was waiting outside to pick me up, which was true, and I was fired. I'm sure my boss just needed an excuse to get rid of me.

After my bakery working experiment, I told my parents I wanted to try living on my own for a while and rented a small cabin on a site with eight or ten other cabins very near to where my parents had their store before they moved to the country property. Brock, whose red hair was wild and thinning and was probably in his late 60's, was the owner of the cabins and service station and lived in a house on the cabins property. He gave me a job pumping gas, checking oil and washing windshields, and if anybody asked, I would also check the tire pressure. So basically, doing the long-lost art of full service. I can still remember that diesel fuel at the time was a lot cheaper than regular gas but not so nowadays. One afternoon after I got home, I heard a knock at my door. It was a young woman from a few cabins over asking to borrow a can opener. I gave her mine to use and closed the door. A few moments later I got another knock at the door. This time it was Brock, inebriated, who asked if he could come in.

As he sat down, he started telling me to be careful of the young woman as she had been knocking at my door several times that day while I was at work. He went on to say that if she came into my cabin for sex that I should throw my wallet under the bed so she couldn't steal my money. At first, I thought it was very sound advice but then again, I laughed to myself. How often is he looking at my cabin? And why? He also told me that, if I wanted, I could have his boots and he began taking them off. I pleaded "But, I don't want your boots." and he put them back on and left. I enjoyed living on my own with the proud feeling of being somewhat independent, but Brock was a heavy drinker and would become unpredictable at times yelling at me for what seemed to be no reason. This made me nervous and on edge wondering what was coming next. One night, not very late, some friends of mine dropped me off and just beeped a very short beep on the horn as they were leaving. Brock came out of his house yelling at me for making so much noise. I had enough walking on eggshells, so the next morning I went to his house and told him I quit and that I was moving out. I moved back home.

GOLF ANYONE?

In the summer of 1974, 16 years old, underage, I was at a local bar with a friend when a couple of girls I knew came to our table asking for a ride home. My friend Randy was driving, and he said no problem. The bar was closing so Randy and I went up to the girls who were sitting at a table with a bunch of guys, telling the girls we were ready to go. One of the guys at the table put cigarette ashes on my pants as I was crouching down but I just ignored it. We headed outside with the girls behind us, the guys following us out as well. They were driving beside us, 3 guys in the front of their car, and 3 in the back and were swerving at us back-and-forth trying to run us off the road. At one point one of the guys was hanging out of their window trying to open our gas cap and then mooned us. We dropped the girls off, but the other car had followed us purposely blocking us in. We were trapped and it didn't feel like it was going to end well. A chill ran up my spine. Randy and I had been golfing that day, so we pulled out our clubs to protect ourselves. One guy grabbed my club out of my hand and started swinging, grazing me with it. I grabbed the club back and smashed their back window. They smashed part of our windshield and took off but stopped again down the street. We left and they were following us again. We stopped at a red light and one guy got out of the other car, drop kicked my window but didn't break it. They were blocking us again, so furious at this point I got out and broke their front window and headlights with a club. One of the guys grabbed a club, a nine iron, and hit me a couple times in the back, then losing his grip, I got the club back, and I got him a couple times. I didn't know where Randy was, but looked way up the street about a block and saw a silhouette of Randy chasing a guy with a club. Randy came back, they got back in their car, and we got in ours. Randy and I went to the police who brought the others in. We were told we were all were in the wrong and we might as well just forget about it.

During the summer of 1975, I decided to try and get a job in Winnipeg. At the time, I worked at the big bakery in Thunder Bay and I had bought a new colour TV. Since I was going to Winnipeg to try and find work, my parents bought the TV from me to try and help me out with some money. With only a suitcase full of clothes and my CB radio, I hitched a ride with a truck driver arriving in Winnipeg after a ten hour or so drive. He dropped me off at a hotel by the airport called The Airliner and I got a room for the night. During the evening, I went downstairs to the lobby to buy a little snack from a vending machine, and then returned to my room. After a few moments, my heart started to race when I realised that my wallet was missing. In a panic, I hurried back to the lobby to try and find it. I was looking all over including under the seat cushions of a sofa that I had sat on for a few minutes. Just then, the concierge noticed my looking for something and asked me what I was doing. I told him about the wallet and after he asked me my name, he handed my wallet back to me. I had left it on top of the candy machine. I was so relieved that I kept thanking him as I walked away. Early the next morning, I plugged in my CB radio but with no antennae I had no signal and couldn't hear anyone. I decided to improvise and took a metal clothes hanger from the closet and with a piece of speaker wire hooked it all up. Within a few minutes I was already talking to other radio people and told one guy that I needed a place to stay and that I was looking for work. A few hours later we met, and he took me back to his house where I could stay in the spare bedroom. I spent about a week looking for a band or any other work, but really spent a lot of time lying in bed listening to my music from some tapes and an 8-track player I had with me. I was rocking myself for hours every day so full of anxiety. I decided to go back to Thunder Bay and through my new friend was set up with a ride home with a truck driver.

In 1975 through early 1976 (like a lot of people) I was into citizens band (CB) radio. Basically, people had radios that they could talk to each other on across distances. Through the radio a group of people got to know each other over the airwaves and later hung out together from time to time. I made a lot of new friends, and it was really a lot of fun. There was one mouthy teenager who kept harassing some of the CBers. One night it was decided that we were going to cut his cable that ran from the radio to the antenna outside. There was a group of five or six of us that left in two vehicles to go do this; I was in a jeep. We got to the kid's place who was still on the radio at that time. It was the perfect moment. We snuck into his backyard and with somebody quietly lifting me up to get as much cable as possible, we cut a big piece and went running back to the vehicles. It was wintertime and I was only wearing regular shoes not boots, I slipped under the jeep cutting my leg quite badly on the undercarriage. It hurt like crazy taking the breath out of me. We quickly got into our vehicles, left and a few minutes later the kid came back on the radio from next-door to his place saying that he saw who did it and we better admit it, or he was going to call the police. We knew he was bluffng. We went to the jeep drivers' home where they patched up my left leg (I should've had stitches), and I still carry a very big scar because of this. The mouthy kid never found out who it was that did the cutting and he toned down his attitude quite a bit.

THE BAND YEARS

After trying several types of jobs in Thunder Bay in 1976, I ended up going to the Community College to study electronics repair. I was six months into the one-year course when one of the students told me he might know of a job for me with a travelling band playing in Nipigon where he lived. It was a band from Toronto called The Richard Gordon Revue who were looking for a drummer. I found that prospect exciting and said I was interested. He gave them my number and they called that evening but they were so desperate I was hired without an audition. They picked me up with my drums, and off we went to Sioux Lookout, a small-town west of Thunder Bay. After the several hour highway drive and then another few hours driving off the highway, we arrived the night before playing and asked a passerby where the bar was. The girl said "Oh! you must be the band!" (I guess they didn't get many tourists there). The next afternoon we set up our equipment and went over a few of the songs on stage which we were going to play that night. I was elated and beyond excited. After playing about three or four songs, the leader of the band, Gord, said to the rest of the band "He's not much, but he's all we've got." While that comment stunned me and knocked me down a few pegs, it helped me to realize that I wasn't really all that good yet. Ray, the sax player was a great mentor to me as he would practice several hours every day, which set a great example for me to follow. During my 3 months with this band, I started practicing many hours each day which I would continue doing for years. I became very dedicated and would play with a band 4 hours a night waiting for the club to close at one o'clock in the morning, then practice while the cleaners worked. I'd continue to work on many styles and rhythms till about 4 in the morning, teaching myself how to read drum charts. I'd go to bed, get up around noon and practice till about 2 in the afternoon in our room with a scaled down version of my drums. I used towels on top of the drums to deaden the sound. I'd have dinner around 5 o'clock and after dinner practice for a couple more hours. This became my routine for about 5 years with several bands while on the road. Years earlier, as a child, I had taken piano lessons for 2 years.

Many times, I needed to work in Thunder Bay at the family greenhouses from winter to spring to make enough money to go back and live in Toronto. After a long day working I'd go into the soil shed where my drums were set up and practice for three or four hours. The shed wasn't heated so my Mom bought me a little heater to use while practicing. I'd pile boxes six feet high all the way around my drum set and put a cover of greenhouse plastic on top of the boxes which kept the warmness from the heater in. For a couple of years while on the road, I took my digital metronome and put it under my pillow at night to try and help myself feel steady timing and improve my drumming. I'd start out very slow, each night increasing the pulse by two beats a minute until many days later it was set at the fastest tempo. I'd then go back to the slowest again. I'd go to sleep like this and wake up in the morning refreshed and feeling the beat. I'd also practice my drumming along with music while wearing headphones. I worked at it a lot. In Gord's band, I was seventeen years old (I probably looked more like thirteen years old), but told them I was eighteen, which was the drinking age at that time. I believe now that Gord (who was also a very talented artist) knew I was underage as every day he would black pencil in my thin little moustache to make me look older. It was during my time with this band that I started calling my Mom every Sunday, something I continued to do for many years. My Mom knew that if she didn't hear from me for a few weeks that I wasn't doing well and had probably quit a band or been fired. I just didn't want to call and burden her with my problems when things weren't going great.

At one bar where The Richard Gordon Revue played in Fort Frances Ontario, the owner asked me several times how old I "really" was. I just kept repeating "eighteen, going to be nineteen". He would reply "are you sure it's not seventeen going to be eighteen?" Soon after, I would just start telling people I was twenty years old, I was always a little afraid of my actual age being found out.

At another gig, we were playing a very fast song where the dancers were on the same level as the stage. They were whipping each other around; I wasn't watching and next thing I knew I got the surprise of being under my drums with a shocked lady on top of the pile. Both a little startled we helped each other up. She said she'd pay for any damage which at first there didn't appear to be any because of the lack of good lighting in the bar. I told her not to worry about it, a few days later noticing a big crack in one of the Tom Toms. These red drums were made of acrylic, so I used a little crazy glue fixing it up almost like new.

When we played in Brandon, Manitoba not far from Winnipeg, I met Ding, a Malaysian woman who was three years older than me. We hit it off well and hung out together for the three weeks while our band was playing at the bar. On the last day of our gig, she was in my room and said to me "I'm coming with you" I asked her what she meant. "I'm quitting my studies at the University and coming with you." She replied. I agreed with her plan, unfortunately for her and her studies. I was very young and immature at the time and didn't understand the ramifications of what she had done by coming with me. Her family was not happy and after travelling with me for several weeks her sister told her on the phone that she had to come back to Manitoba, having violated being sponsored in Canada. I was very worried about what might happen to Ding and recommended that she return. After further conversations with her sister, Ding told me that it would be better if she just went back to Malaysia via Winnipeg. I felt terrible about the situation I had put her in. Ray, the Sax player, and I ended up quitting the band and went to Winnipeg to look for work, bringing Ding with us on a bus. I didn't even have the courage to go to the airport with her. Ding and I said our goodbyes in Winnipeg at the hotel Ray and I were staying at. She left in a cab and that's the last time I ever saw her. We kept in touch for about six months, I sent her a letter telling her when she gets back to Canada on her own maybe we could get a place together. I never heard from her again. I had tried many times over the years to contact her always feeling quite a bit of guilt and wanting to know that things turned out well for her. I never got a reply. I hope that life treated her well even though she had left her studies. Her family owned a large sugar factory in Kuala Lumpur so they may have been able to help her financially.

Ray and I stayed in Winnipeg for about a week or so looking for a gig, but we couldn't find a full-time band that was looking for a drummer or saxophonist. He offered to take me to Toronto where he was renting a room in an apartment from some friends of his, a couple named Rick and Brenda. Coming from a small town and even though the biggest city I had been in at that point was Winnipeg, I decided to take him up on his offer and go. I didn't know what to expect. We left for Toronto on a bus arriving on that summer evening after traveling for about twenty eight hours. A few hours after settling in the apartment in Scarbourough, a suburb of Toronto, Rick who I thought looked like a beatnik with his black stringy long beard and hair, arrived home from work. He looked me over as if to ask, "What are you doing here?", especially since I was sitting in his Captain's chair. Ray quietly told me "That's Ricks chair.". So naive and wondering what the big deal was I got out of the chair and turned in early that night, sleeping on the floor, Ray on a piece of foam, knowing that I wasn't exactly welcomed with open arms.

The next day in my new city I decided I was going to go to The Entertainer's Contact Service which was located uptown. I could see the CN Tower building downtown from the window of the apartment and thought it didn't look too far. Wide eyed and inexperienced in a big city, I started out that day walking and walking and walking and walking not realizing that uptown was about 10 miles away. I kept asking people along the way how far the address I was heading to was. Some would say "You're walking it? why don't you just take the bus?"

Undaunted, I kept going, arriving hours later and signing up for the service. I auditioned for a couple of bands through them but never did get any work having better success over the years putting my own ad in the 'dramatic musical talent' section of the Toronto Star newspaper where I could be very specific about what I was looking for. Several days after my arrival, I was told by Rick that I couldn't stay there any longer and would have to leave. Rick and his wife Brenda weren't happy at all with me being there. Feeling so unwanted I called the bass player from Gord's band and asked him if I could stay at his place. The answer was emphatically "no." Coming from a small town and being naive, I assumed that everybody was going to look out for me. A few days later after talking to Rick and Brenda about it for a while they did agree to let me stay. Very relieved, I was able to buy my own humble piece of foam and not be sleeping on the hard floor anymore. The sax player moved out a year later, with me staying on till around 1981. During my stay, Rick owned a pile of different types of guns and ammo, so I made sure I always paid my rent on time.

Late one night, he took me downtown in his souped-up 1927 Model T Ford. Heading south down Yonge Street on the main strip all eyes were on us and the car as we drove by. Rick floored it. At first the car went left a little bit and then right a little bit and then straight ahead like a rocket for about six blocks. Man, that car was fast. Rick obviously was not worried if the police would see us.

During my first six months while living at the apartment, I took a job at Zing Burger, a local eatery. Before I got the job, I was broke. I was spending a lot of time in bed rocking myself and hadn't eaten for several days. Every day I would look at the classifieds in the newspaper with every intention of applying for work but mentally I just couldn't do it, even showing up at businesses to apply but not going inside. One day, I went into Zing Burger to buy something to drink with the little bit of cash I had and struck up a conversation with Len, one of the young cooks. In conversation, I told him I didn't have money for food and had not eaten for a while. I was just telling what was going on and wasn't trying to get a free meal. Out of the kindness of his heart, he made me a free steak sandwich, which I devoured. I was very thankful. A few days later I saw the help wanted sign in Zing Burger's window, applied, and got hired.

There was a young kid named Manny who worked there who had his name and telephone number and the words "call me" on his T-shirt. I never did ask him if he got any calls. Sometimes after working till closing time, Len, Joe, and I would drive to Buffalo New York for breakfast, the first trip arriving with only Canadian money. That time, the waitress looked at me like I had three heads when I asked if they took Canadian money, surprising me that it wasn't accepted at the restaurant. We had to return to Toronto hungry, the next trips all of us bringing some American cash.

One day, a customer was unhappy with the way his burger was cooked and brought it back to Joe. The customer told Joe to "fire it" meaning put it back on the grill. Joe pointed at the burger and said "you're fired!' and walked away. I really enjoyed working at Zing Burger and stayed on for about six months eventually auditioning for bands again after feeling well enough to do so.

No cake for you!

I left Zing Burger to take a job with a band called Lodestar. We rehearsed for a couple of weeks and went on the road to our first job in Kapuskasing in Northern Ontario. We were booked at that bar for two weeks arriving late in the afternoon on the first day. We set up our equipment to play later that evening still having a little bit of time to spare. I was going to go for an hour nap upstairs in my room but as I walked down the hallway some guy came out of his room and asked me to come and have a drink with him. I told him that we had just arrived, and I was just going to have a nap, but he very much insisted. I eventually gave in and went to his room to have a drink. I sat down and he poured a drink that was about half a litre by the looks of it into a large glass. I didn't take a sip yet as he turned around and started playing very strange sounding music on his cassette player. I also had an uneasy feeling about the things he was saying and went to get up out of the chair to leave. He grabbed me by the shoulder and pushed me back down and said, "You're not going fucking anywhere." I didn't know what the guy wanted but I wasn't about to hang around to find out. He turned around preoccupied while attending to the music, so I headed out the door walking very fast down the hallway. He came running out to the hallway shouting "I've got a gun you better come back!" which made me walk even faster. I went downstairs shaking and told the band about it and we decided to call the police. The OPP (Provincial Police) came to talk to me for a few minutes and basically just said "the guy is okay, we know him, and he 'probably' doesn't have a gun." That night we played for the crowd and the guy was in the audience staring at me the whole time from the bar. I was feeling very uneasy but tried my best to keep my composure and concentrate on the music. I would find out later after leaving that gig from one of the band members that they had gone to his room that night, had a drink with the guy, and were shown his gun.

Later in the week it was my birthday and the bass player had given me a nice card and a six pack of Heineken. At that point I had only worked with the band for a couple weeks, so I thought that was pretty nice thing to do. That night during the first set, the lights dimmed, and someone carrying a cake with lit candles was making their way to the front of the stage. The leader of the band said, "It's Keith's birthday, come on up to the front Keith!" As I got to the front of the stage, I went to blow the candles out when from behind me Henry, the bass player forcefully stuck a big pie in my face, which not only got me but was all over my drums. At first, I thought it was the cake that had been pushed into my face and was frantically trying to get the lit candles off, then realising that it was only a pie and not the cake. I laughed about it with only my pride a little damaged, not the drums. I cleaned them off and finished out the week. I was so relieved when we left that place still thinking about the story of the man with the gun that the guys in the band told me. I don't know if they were telling me that as a joke or if it was for real.

During this time in my life I was often spending the afternoons privately rocking away on the bed. The lead guitar player asked me one day what I was doing listening to music with the lights off and curtains drawn. Of course, I was embarrassed and did that so no one could see what I was doing, I just couldn't tell him that. This band only stayed together for four weeks. The lead guitar player in this band went on to have a very succesful carreer in film and Television composing.

Angus Walker

Back in Toronto, I had an advertisement in the Toronto Star newspaper looking for a band and received a call from Angus Walker a country artist who was playing in Saint-Georges-de-Malbaie, Quebec. I agreed that I would travel the 1500 kilometers (932 miles) to audition, putting all my drums on a bus before heading out.

It was a long trip, and I was really exhausted by the time we arrived, having at first missed my stop and gone past the hotel by a couple of miles. I unloaded my drums from the bus, leaving them on the side of the road, being lucky enough to have someone passing by with a pick-up truck give me a ride with all my equipment to the hotel. I auditioned and got the gig which was great since I didn't have any money with which to go back to Toronto.

While playing at that bar I developed a drinking problem. I would wake up in the morning with my case of beer beside me on the floor. Before I got out of bed I would drink two bottles, drink all day before work, then have four or five beers at the club. I guess I must have gotten used to it because I wasn't really hammered at any time. I wasn't sober, but I wasn't drunk either, all during the six months I played with this band. I eventually stopped drinking completely for a couple years.

When I did go back to drinking, I was doing it in moderation. It was more that I was not well mentally at the time and was self-medicating with alcohol. Years later, I was told by a psychiatrist that this indeed had been the case.

Angus had a nickname for me which was Herk (short for Hercules because I was so skinny at 5 feet, 10 inches tall and weighed 130 pounds). I accepted that nickname with a little bit of pride. While travelling the East Coast with the band for several months we played in Prince Edward Island. While there I met a lovely young girl named Loretta. I was nineteen she was only seventeen and we really hit it off. She was living with family at the time including four sisters, two brothers, and her Father (her Mother having passed away years before during childbirth). I travelled more on the road but would always visit her on the weekends, taking the ferry across the water with the guitar player (Frank) in our band whose girlfriend also lived there.

During one winter weekend visit on Prince Edward Island, we were leaving in Frank's blue Volkswagen on the Monday to travel to play our first night that evening in Nova Scotia. We got stuck in a snowstorm, were already over an hour late and still trying to make our way to the gig. After trying to find the bar for a while, we had gotten close but it was still across lanes of highway and snowbanks. We were on the wrong side not being able to figure out how to get on the correct lane to turn into driveway. After a brief deliberation we decided to leave the car on the side of the highway and walk across all the lanes and ditches in knee deep snow. When we finally got across to the bar, Angus met us at the door and said, "If the owner asks, tell him you were in a car accident because that's what I told him." Actually, Frank and I had been in a car accident in Halifax a week or so earlier and the front end of the car did have a big dent. Angus and Don, the bass player, had set up my drums and I laughed and wondered at the time if they had ever done that before as the whole setup was backwards. After readjusting my drums and everyone tuning up, we played the remaining part of that evening and the rest of the week.

Eventually, being on the road was not great for our relationship and Loretta and I stopped seeing each other.

I continued to work with Angus for a couple more months even playing drums in a studio on four of his original songs. Eventually, I wanted to leave the band because Don, the bass player and I weren't getting along, and I wanted to audition for bands that weren't playing country music. The arguments became a pattern, following me from band to band and many other parts of my life. My mental state always had me on the defensive, as well, I always felt like I had to prove myself and that people were out to get me. Angus and the band were heading to Toronto, and I got a ride back to the city with Frank. It was late at night when we arrived in Toronto so I took most of my stuff out of his car planning to get the rest the following day. The next day I called the number where Frank was staying, but he had left for Sarnia with all my music L.P's, an expensive bass drum pedal, a radio/tape player, all my tax receipts for that year and a few other things. It's amazing that

I can still remember what was in the car, but at the time it was pretty much all I had. I picked up my drums from Angus' van whom I wasn't in touch with again for many years. I never did get any of my stuff back from Frank, even calling his parents several months later to inquire about it. In 2015 Angus and I reconnected and are still in touch regularly. In the time I worked with him, I looked up to him as a father figure. He always treated me very well and I respected him. Don and I reconnected as well and were friends again up until he passed away.

Heather Haig

From around the age of 15, I had asthma and was going through a lot of stressful situations in my life. I made many trips to the Hospital's emergency department telling them I couldn't breathe, one time asking my Dad to take me saying I needed to know if I was going to die or not. My Dad said sadly to me in Dutch "*kint*," which is "child" in English. I could see he was frustrated with me. Obviously I was mentally not well, a hypochondriac and the staff at the emergency department started to get to recognise me.

At age twenty, when I worked with Heather Haig, the whole band (including our manager) were living in his house together. One night I was having a severe panic attack and again was having breathing problems. George, our manager took me to the hospital. We were sitting in the emergency waiting room, but things were not moving fast enough. I started to hyperventilate even more and fell to the floor. The alarm bells went off and the staff came, picked me up and brought me in having me breathe into a paper bag for a few minutes. After I calmed down, I was able to breath normally again. They told me it was psychosomatic and asked George if he was my father. Later in my mid-twenties, I learned how to channel my anxiety and stress by using slow deep breathing techniques and reading positive affirmation books. The asthma has mostly gone away even to this day. I would stay with Heather's band for a few more months though we really didn't work that much, and I couldn't afford to be off work for weeks at a time. I was broke and still owed a thousand dollars on my drums which my parents paid off plus getting me a bus ticket back to Thunder Bay so I could work at the greenhouses during the busy season from winter to spring. After the season was over, I was still really missing Loretta and decided to go back to Prince Edward Island and find work there. Every time after finishing working the busy season at the greenhouses Mom would be in tears when I would leave, pleading with me to stay in Thunder Bay. I know that my parents didn't want me to have a hard life and they were becoming more and more aware of my struggles. Now, I was moving to Prince Edward Island.

Oh, Those Pancakes!

Getting back to Prince Edward Island in mid spring I immediately put an advertisement in the paper saying, "Young man from Toronto looking for work in Prince Edward Island." I couldn't believe all the responses that I got. So many phone calls! I had offers for a Job in everything from construction to sales. My first job was at a restaurant near the airport. When I went to apply, they asked me if I had cooking experience but I had only worked at the burger place. I said I had worked at Swiss Chalet in Toronto. Not true. I just needed a job so badly and I thought, "really, how hard can it be to cook?" The next day they had me learn where everything was in the kitchen during the training and was told that I was going to be on my own the following day. I kind of swallowed hard for a moment. I still had a lot of nerve and thought I should be okay, going in for my shift at 5:30 am. After about an hour of getting everything prepared, turning on the deep fryer and grill, I thought I was ready to go. An hour later, two tour busses arrived with about seventy-five hungry people on board. I thought "okay, so this is how it's all going to end."

Everyone wanted breakfast! The orders were coming in. There were pancake orders, sandwiches, eggs, everything. In my haste to get the orders out, I kept breaking the yolks on the grill. I put another on and broke the yolk repeat, repeat, sticking the broken ones in the little garbage chute on the grill until the chute was full. At that point one of the waitresses walked in, looked at me for a moment, shook her head, and walked out. I could feel my face was flushed, I felt like I was in a daze. I kept trying though, putting pancakes on which turned into about 14-inches round spreading out on the grill. I found out later I didn't have the grill hot enough and I had added water not milk to them. I was a mess mentally with all the pressure, but I kept pushing through. I eventually got all the orders out. One of the waitresses came in and said to me "About those pancakes…" (I was waiting for the hammer to fall). She said, "The guy said, they were the best damn pancakes he ever had!" I couldn't believe it! With great relief on my part and probably also for the waitresses, the day finally ended, and I went home to Loretta's. I was a little apprehensive about going in to work the next day, but since I had bought a bike to travel to and from home already, I rode it to work for my second morning. I was called into the owner's office. She said, "I heard you had a little trouble yesterday." I said "Yeah, I think I was a little rusty."

I hoped that there was some way I could wiggle out of all this trouble and keep my job. Somehow the owner seemed to accept my answers and I stayed on for another two months, getting my timing down for cooking until I decided I needed a job with less pressure. In pressure situations, I would go blank and not be able to focus at all.

My second job was working at a submarine place downtown that as well as being an enjoyable place to work, had a jukebox I really enjoyed playing. It was a very busy place where we made a lot of the submarines prepared with basic ingredients ahead of time for the lunch crowd or later in the evening for the bar rush. The brother of the owner was not a great guy and was not very nice to any of the staff when the owner wasn't around. One day he came in and was upset that I hadn't taken the garbage out yet. The problem being the garbage can outside the front of the store was full of wasps, hundreds of them. He got upset with me and went out with a can of gas pouring it down the garbage lighting it on fire. The flames were about 4 feet high and within minutes the big window in the front of the store cracked from the heat. When the owner came in, he was wasn't pleased at all and told his brother off who never said another word to me, but because of this tension I quit that job.

I moved on to a job at a restaurant in old Charlottetown being hired as the sous chef, not knowing the man who was the chef wasn't exactly reliable. The first day that I worked with him, I realized he had a bottle of booze in the garbage covered with lettuce leaves. I was a little shocked that he kept taking big swigs from it throughout the day, each time offering for me to join him for a drink. Of course I didn't want to drink on the job knowing that he just wanted me to be doing it with him so I couldn't say anything about him to anyone. I only lasted a few weeks there. That was the last job I had in Prince Edward Island. I missed the music business so much and asked Loretta to come back to Toronto with me which she declined not wanting to leave her family behind. A few days later I left the island.

One of Loretta's brothers who was about twelve years old at the time, and was an aspiring musician, had told me that he was doubting his chances of ever getting into a band himself. I told him at the time that he could accomplish anything he set his mind to by working hard on it. Seventeen years later, I returned to Prince Edward Island for a visit and had a conversation with the brother who was now a successful leader of a band playing all over the east coast. He brought up our conversation (which I had completely forgotten) and said it really helped him apply himself and kept him practicing and believing in himself over the years. I had no idea that my words could have influenced someone in this way. It was a very humbling moment.

TORONTO, HOME AGAIN

Upon returning to Toronto, I auditioned for several bands including The Stampeders (they were expanding the band with keyboards and horns and Kim Berly the drummer/vocalist was going to front the band I think). There was a huge drum kit set up, way bigger than I ever owned, I was a little intimidated and nervous and didn't get the job.

Sweet Surrender

My next audition was for Sweet Surrender, a show band playing disco, funk, rock 'n' roll and contemporary rock. I got the gig and since we were rehearsing in the same building, I happened to bump into the drummer from The Stampeders in the hallway. He said "Hi! more auditions?" I replied "No, I've got a gig, we're rehearsing down the hall." He looked a little surprised as I had only auditioned for them just a few days before. I wasn't one to wait around in those days, auditioning when I could. At twenty-one years old, my drumming had gotten to the point where I was good enough to work in music styles that I preferred. When I first joined Sweet Surrender we only had one lead singer Barrie, Murphy on keyboards, me on drums, Albert on bass and Lonnie on guitar. We also had a soundman who owned all the sound equipment (speakers, microphones and truck). I remember playing one club just outside of Toronto that had put an advertisement in the paper saying Sweet Surrender was playing and that "they have a million dollars worth of equipment that is taking up half the room." At first, we were playing in Toronto and surrounding areas as well as northern Ontario.

While playing in Wawa, Ontario I had a fight with our bass player. We were all drinking in our chalet and I pulled all the drawers out of his dresser, spilling all the clothes on the floor. I don't know why I did that; I guess at the time I thought it was funny, but nobody else was laughing. Albert pushed me to the floor and started choking me. As I was blacking out, he stopped, stood up, and shouted, "Hit me …hit me!" so I hit him, and that's when Barrie and Lonnie got between us and broke up the fight. Out of breath, I sat down on a chair, holding my foot and felt some wetness on my sock. I looked at my hand and it was covered in blood; I had stepped on a broken beer bottle. I thought, what do I do now? We both ended up going to the local hospital, I had five stitches and Albert got a little brace on his nose, it was not broken. I played the rest of the week on crutches and with stitches in my bass drum foot. This caused me to only be able to press the pedal very gingerly, leaving the soundman turning the sound up as high as he could for the drum so that the audience could hear it. We ended up getting rid of the soundman not too long after and instead hired a girl singer up front in his place, which meant we also had to rent a truck and sound equipment. Apparently, we could get a lot more work that way.

We auditioned many singers and settled on Janet, playing mostly major and medium sized cities including Toronto, Southern Ontario then out West. After starting a tour in Winnipeg, we were on our way to Regina to a club called The Old Gold. We got about halfway there, were running out gas, and it was -30 c outside. Luckily, we had enough gas to just make it to a service station which was closed as it was late, around 3 am. Barrie got on the payphone and called the local police to help us. The police called the garage owner, got him out of bed and had him come and open up and give us gas. He was not too happy as by then it was four o'clock in the morning. We had completely run out of gas and were sitting in the cold truck by the time the owner got to us. It was so fortunate that we made it to his station and that we didn't freeze to death on the road somewhere. With this band and many others I worked with traveling across Canada we slept when we could, often on large speakers or in-between luggage.

Another of our bookings was at a Chinese

restaurant and bar in downtown Calgary called Pons Palace. I remember Barrie saying to the crowd which was a dinner crowd and we were a very loud show band "We're going to start off with some slow quiet music and then blow the wontons into your face during the second set." Everybody in the band laughed but we weren't sure how the audience took it because we couldn't see them for the stage lights that were shining in our faces.

Another night after leaving the bar and walking through the kitchen Barrie made some kind of wise crack comment to the Chinese cook chopping up chicken with a meat cleaver. The cook looked up, slammed the cleaver into the chicken and said "Oh! you wanna be a chic-kon?" Mostly, Barrie thought of himself as funny but sometimes he would go too far.

Most of the gigs out west were two to three weeks long. We also played a club in Saskatoon called Fast Freddy's. We were always working on new music and would practice during the day at whatever club we were booked at. One morning as we arrived at the club to rehearse, we realized no one was there and the door was locked. Barrie got the great idea (he thought anyway) to jimmy the lock so we could get in to rehearse so he did just that. We were there for about an hour when the cook showed up, kind of looked us over but went into the kitchen. A half hour after that the club owner showed up and asked Barrie "how did you guys get in here?" Barrie just made a bunch of vague excuses of how we managed to get in. The club owner walked away shaking his head. Of course, Barrie never did come clean and tell him we broke in.

It was an interesting group of people in this band. Murphy the keyboard player would sleep with one eye open which was rather unnerving especially since I was rooming with him and never really knew if he was asleep or just watching me. About four months into the tour the lead singers Barrie and Janet who were involved in a relationship were arguing most of the time especially early in the morning which would wake us all up. It was getting to be too much for everybody in the band, I had enough, quit, and caught a train from out west with my drums back to Toronto.

G.G. Gibson

I was in a show band playing funk, and Caribbean music that had several incarnations with mostly different musicians, G.G. and I being the mainstays. This particular band was practising in Toronto, and had some gigs booked with a new keyboard player, a bass player (Delroy) and guitar player (Rick). The bass player was obviously having some mental difficulties and was saying some very strange things during rehearsals which raised everybody's eyebrows. I didn't know anything about schizophrenia at that time although now I would say that's probably what was going on with him. We were originally rehearsing with a different bass player, but he had wanted to bring some girls on the road to work in the hotels for him. There was no way G.G. was going to bring a pimp/bass player with us. After a couple of weeks practicing with the new bass player, we left for Quebec City. The new keyboard player said he was going to make his own way to the gig, the rest of us were travelling there in a rented Winnebago. During the drive, Delroy kept pointing up to the lights and rubbing his fingers on one hand, with me having no idea what was going through his mind. I finally asked, "what are you doing?" and he replied "greens!" That still didn't answer my question. On the road some bands I worked with would play word games to make the miles seem to pass faster. Someone would start with the letter A and name a band starting with that letter. The next person would also have to come up with a name of a band starting with A and then move on to B when A was exhausted and so on. We'd go through the alphabet and when someone would get stumped, they would be out of the game. We'd also do this with movies. Once we finally got to Quebec and were setting up, Delroy wanted to put his amp facing the wall instead of out toward the crowd. He said it would sound better. I'm not sure if it would actually sound better but G.G refused to let him do it which made Delroy very angry.

After we had finished setting up, we went to the band house where we would be sleeping and eating during the gig. I was tired and planned on catching an hour nap before the show. A short while later, I was abruptly awakened from a deep sleep hearing Rick yelling "Keith, it's Delroy, he's got a knife and is going for GG." I ran out into the hall not sure what was going on and confronted Delroy punching him once and getting him to drop the knife. He wanted to know what I did that for as he claimed he was just going to make a sandwich. I said "Yeah, out of G.G.!"

We got to the club a couple hours before we we're going to play, and the keyboard player hadn't shown up yet. I said to G.G. "give me his number, I'll give him a call," hoping that he was already on his way. When he answered the phone still in Toronto, and us in Quebec City, I knew that was not a good thing. I asked, "when are you coming here?" He said, "I'll try and come tomorrow". I thought, "he's going to try?" I hung up the phone. We played the first set without the keyboard player. Delroy was an excellent bass player but was obviously not well. During the first break, he threatened the owner of the club who told us at the end of the night that if we wanted to play the next night, we would have to get another bass player. Considering we'd have to rehearse with somebody new and we didn't have the keyboard player, we talked it over and decided to forfeit the job and get paid for the one night. None of us wanted to travel back to Toronto with Delroy as he was so unpredictable, so we called the police, told them all that had happened, and they had him temporarily arrested on some charge. After being back in Toronto for a few days, Delroy called me looking for his equipment which we had packed up and brought home for him. I told him where it was so he could pick it up. He was completely unaware of anything that had happened in Quebec and certainly was not mad at any of us.

Another version of G.G's band I worked with consisted of a bass player, female singer and guitar player all from Newark New Jersey, G.G, a female singer from New Brunswick and me. One night during our perfomance Don, the bass player was leaning on his amplifier the whole evening. Later, I told Don that if he couldn't be professional he should get out of the music business. He was a huge, muscular guy that had only days earlier confided in me that he had shot someone in Newark as part of a gang ritual. Don came towards me saying, "you better put me out of the music business!" I knew that if things escalated it wasn't going to go well for me so I asked him to sit down so we could talk about it. I apologised but our working relationship was strained after this incident.

I had been keeping a diary in the 1970's to the early 1980's. I was embarrassed and shocked as to what I was reading on paper when I went back and read it all from the beginning. That day, I burned it, not being able to handle seeing my life laid out before me in that way. I had been a womanizer, argumentative, combative, and really couldn't get along with anybody in my working and personal life. I had some idea how very bad I had gotten but reading it in print was distressing to me and I didn't want to be the person in that diary. I wasn't a particularly nice person, and it was evident to me now how unwell mentally I really was all those years. Even dating back to my childhood, early teens and later in my twenties I was unwell, having gotten into many fist fights and arguments.

During one winter through spring in the 1980's, I lived in the east end of Montreal with my girlfriend who was a hairstylist downtown. Some nights, I would buy a six pack of beer at the corner store near her apartment. I had become friendly with the owner who seemed like a nice enough guy, maybe 60 years old, and was tall and slim. He was a character and I would often leave the store laughing. Late one evening I was making a run to the store and the owner was waiting by the door, this time standing with a silver pistol tucked into his waist band. He said in his "chantant" (sing songy) French-Canadian accent, "They robbed me last night but tonight I'm ready for them." It all made me a little nervous, the gun and everything. I don't know why, but I still got my six pack of beer. I paid for it, and never went back.

The owners of the hair place where my girlfriend worked seemed very unscrupulous being involved in crimes including drugs. They invited us both to a "party" one night which consisted of only two guys from her work and the two of us. I was naive and clueless that this could be any kind of trouble. When we got to their house, I could plainly see it was full of all kinds of products like TVs, VCRs, microwaves and rolled up carpets.

We all were drinking quite heavily. Being inebriated, I thought I was having a good time relaxing, not really paying attention. I noticed my girlfriend and the younger guy were laughing while walking into another room, with me thinking they were just going into the kitchen. The older fellow said to me "You don't mind that he's fucking your girlfriend?" I said "What are you talking about?" So, he expanded "She's in the room with him now near the kitchen." I went to the room where they were in and tried to open the door, but something was holding it closed. I forced the door open to find the guy was standing naked just inside the door. He started yelling "What are you doing? she wanted it!" He shouted that about three times. I was so upset I sucker punched him. My girlfriend, fully clothed grabbed my hand and said, "Let's get out of here!" The guy was slowly putting his clothes back on and said to me "You think you know how to fight? I'll show you how to fight!" Completely immersed in fear we ran out into the street, flagging down a passing bus not sure of exactly where we were. It was in the wee hours of the morning as we made our way back to my girlfriend's apartment. The next day when she got home from work, she told me the guy I punched said he was going to knock me dead the next time he saw me. She also told me that he had been a professional boxer in the past. I ended up leaving Montreal the next day to go back to Toronto. Cowardly, yes, but I had no idea what kind of people I was dealing with or what they were capable of. She and I were never in touch again.

I just couldn't go!

The next summer while I was living in and looking after a couple of musicians friends' apartment downtown while they were playing in Lars, Germany, I discovered that I wasn't able to pee all day long, but I kept waiting and waiting thinking that later it would eventually fix itself. It didn't, so later that night I went to The Wellesley Hospital nearby and was seen by emergency staff. I explained my situation and that I was in a lot of discomfort with a full bladder. They processed me fast, put me in a cubicle and a male nurse took a catheter and tried to pass it through. The catheter would just not go in and the harder he tried, it still wouldn't go, eventually bending the catheter at the middle. He asked me if I'd put something up there (I thought, really?) I found that question to be ridiculous, but they probably saw all kinds of weird things inserted in strange places. Suddenly, when he removed the catheter I started to bleed profusely. I couldn't believe what I was seeing. He started to say while holding onto my penis, "Somethings not right here! somethings not right here!" He left the room, and they phoned a urologist to come in. Before the urologist arrived, I thought maybe I'd be able to go pee, so I went to the washroom. The stream coming out was pure blood instead of urine. It was uncontrollable, I panicked causing the blood to spray all over the wall and toilet. I went out into the hallway pleading, all the while trying to be calm "Help Me! I'm bleeding, I'm bleeding!" They got me back to my bed and the bleeding slowed down again. When the surgeon came in after approximately an hour, it only took him about five minutes to get me opened up again, however before he'd started, he made sure to tell me that he was upset with me for disturbing his dinner date with his girlfriend. I thought to myself, you, buddy, have no idea how much discomfort I was in or how to treat people in a humane way. When the surgeon left, the male nurse came in and apologized to me for making me bleed. They admitted me into the hospital overnight and I ended up staying a couple of days. A doctor at the time told me I have a stricture (in my case, a narrowing of the urethra) but the cause was unknown.

During my hospital stay my sister Bev came by in a clown costume bringing some helium balloons and tied them to my walking pole. This was very cute and thoughtful of her and with her doing clowning quite appropriate. I had the same retention issue about three or four years later and I had to get my urethra opened up again. I've had the same procedure done now over the years eight or nine times, the most recent one in 2022. I had been fine for ten years up to that point and was advised now that I may be good for another ten years, thankfully.

Telling this story reminds me that when I was about 12 years old one of the school bullies came up to me and asked if I had any sleeping bags. I said "Yes, I have two at home" (because we did). He kicked me hard in the groin and yelled "Well then, wake them up!" In excruciating pain, I fell backwards and ended up having to go to the hospital because I couldn't pee the rest of the day. The doctor just said to drink plenty of liquids, and it should fix itself, which it did at that time; I wonder now if that early injury is what caused my problems later. The funny part of that story is that after I got kicked, got home, and told my Mom what happened, Mom, obviously a little uncomfortable with the question asked me "Did you get kicked in the stick or the bag?"

What's your sign? Spiritual Journey

During my mid to late twenties, I read the Gita, Bible, Koran, as well as books on psychology, parapsychology, aliens, and many self-help and other spiritual books. I also was interested in and read a lot of books on astrology and numerology and I was able to do my whole life chart in numerology in the 1980s. I did one for a friend and he did my astrological life chart. It was uncanny how much happened in my life later that was in both charts. I didn't tell him what my numerology chart said until after he did my astrology chart. It was unreal how both predicted many of the same things that could only be unique to my life, my numerology chart saying that I was going to have a serious life altering illness at age thirty, which did happen. The astrology chart was done with the place of my birth, exact time of my birth, day, date and year.

Dockie Roberts

I worked with a number of funk, reggae, and soca bands in the 1980s. Having been out of work I had an ad in the newspaper looking for a gig and got a call from Dockie Roberts who was playing in Regina, Saskatchewan. I flew there along with all my equipment, auditioned, and got the job. I had auditioned for his band several years earlier in Toronto but wasn't a very good player yet and didn't get the job then. I'm not sure if he had remembered that audtion because he never mentioned it. Dockie, the leader and lead singer had an excellent, deep soulful voice. It was a very good soul/funk, disco band with seasoned players and I was very happy to be working with them. We continued for a few more weeks out west and then when the tour was over, we were heading back to Toronto. Before we went through Thunder Bay on our way back the guitar player and bass player were pressing Dockie where the next gig was. Since they questioned Dockie they were both fired and left in Thunder Bay at the train station with all their equipment. That bass player went on to work and record with Billy Idol and Alannah Myles. He and the guitar player are both excellent musicians.

Back in Toronto we started rehearsals after finding two musicians to take their place. We traveled out east with the new version of this band and played about a month in Quebec. In my time with this band, I was very argumentative, and I was playing quite loudly as I couldn't really feel the music at times when the rhythm section wasn't working as a unit. Being still inexperienced I was trying to make up for the lack of groove with playing louder. This wasn't good at all. One night in Quebec after the first set, the band was in the change room, and while I was having an argument with Dockie He said to me "Where have you been man?" (Meaning I hadn't done anything in my life). I said, "It doesn't matter where I've been we're both in the same place now." That comment just infuriated him, he fired me and told me I was going to have to make my own way back to Toronto. His exact words were "Get your ass on the road yourself." He told the members of the band if anybody tried to put my equipment on the truck that they would be staying with me. Worried about not getting paid for the week, I told him that if he wanted me to play the rest of the night, he'd have to pay me right then, which he did, which was great as I had no other money. After the band packed up the equipment and left that night, I went to my room and slept. The next day I got a taxi with all my drums to the train station in the next town, only to find out the train for the day connecting to Toronto had already left. I was disappointed. I was told at the train station that I could leave my drums there overnight. Planning to leave the next day I ended up spending the night at a bed-and-breakfast not far from the station. The owners there were lovely. The room included a free breakfast which I appreciated and enjoyed very much, then made my way back to Toronto once again.

Just Bumming Around

Another winter, broke again, I was back working in Thunder Bay at the greenhouses. My brother John who had taken over the greenhouses around 1977 had added a mini animal farm that had a reindeer, geese, chickens, rabbits and other animals for families to enjoy. We had just gotten in a shipment of about two dozen turkey chicks, but the poor things had a problem. Their little bums were all caked with dried, hard, poop from being transported. It was so bad that they just couldn't poop anymore. Feeling so sorry for those little creatures, I got a Styrofoam coffee cup, some paper towel, some warm water and started to clean their little turkey bums, managing to save them all. That was a feel-good day.

The Directors

Sadly, I have worked with many bands that former members have since passed on. This particular band two of the members that I really admired have recently transitioned: Buzz Thompson (who after the Directors, went on to work with Ronnie Hawkins for many years) and Joe Reynolds, a vibrant singer/trumpet player. It was a good band playing rhythm & blues, soul, and Funk. Both Buzz and Joe had great, soulful voices. We were well received in Toronto and the surrounding towns but not so much in Northern Ontario. We were booked into a rock bar up north where we weren't appreciated at all. During a break one of the girls standing by the door stopped me as I was going outside to get some air and said, "You're the worst band that's ever played here!" (I was actually quite insulted at that comment). As well, some of the guys in the bar used a racial slur in referring to the type of music we were playing and asked why we were playing it being a bunch of white guys.

Coming back from another gig on a beautiful summer day somewhere north of the city, it had been raining heavily that morning and somebody in the band got the idea that we should take a dip in the lake we were passing, which we could easily access from the side of the road. There was a lovely mist over the lake and we started to pull off to the side. As we slowed down the van started to sink deeper and deeper, getting stuck right up to the axle in mud. Many miles from the next town, we were sitting around for an hour wondering what we were going to do. There was very little traffic going by when what a stroke of luck! A pick-up truck with a winch happened by and pulled us out.

One Gig we did was in Sudbury Ontario. We were supposed to play there for two weeks and arrived on time on the Monday and set up our equipment. The first set of the night there were only a couple people in the bar so someone in the band got the idea that we should just have a jam session for the whole set instead of doing our high energy professional show. I could see the lady owner walking around watching us the whole set and then disappeared for a while. After we got off the stage, she informed us that she had called the booking agent and was getting a different band to come in starting Thursday. I wasn't so shocked as the first set was terrible. Since we had that job till Wednesday, we played our hearts out and by Wednesday night the bar was packed. That night, as we started packing after the show, the owner came by and accused us of taking some of the colored light gels that gave the lighting more depth. Those gels were ours and I started to talk back to her saying that she had no right to accuse us, and I couldn't wait to get back to the city. It became a heated argument with her calling me 'city boy' and she left the bar leaving us to finish packing up the rest of the equipment. When we were done, a couple of the band members took a dozen eggs they had and hid them under cushions all over the room thinking they had the last laugh. I'm sure after a few days the bar must have had a very peculiar odor.

True Motion

The guitar player in this band and I disagreed as to who should be keeping the time in the band with him trying to speed the songs up, playing so fast ahead of me that I was trying to fight him to hold back the song tempo. It just sounded terrible. I think it was an ego thing for him and probably for me too, but really, the drummer is supposed to be the timekeeper in the band, otherwise there's just no groove. Over the years, many bands I worked with, the bass player, rhythm guitar and I were a great rhythm section with the drums and bass working together so well that it was rock solid. With True Motion, I remember a week we were playing in Hamilton and a radio station came in and that evening did a live broadcast. Having taped it that night, I listened to the playback to what sounded like me being the worst drummer in the world. The timing for every song was all over the place, speeding up and slowing down.

During the winter we were playing the Holiday Inn in Ottawa. One afternoon while I was in the club tuning my drums, some kid around twenty years old came up to me trying to sell me some cymbal stands and other drum equipment. I wasn't interested and did not have the money to expand my drumkit anyway. It was the end of the last night and we were packing up. I was at the loading dock, it was freezing cold outside, so I went back in to get warmed up and to see how far along we were. I got halfway down the hall and saw a kid walking fast out of the club. At this point it was about 2:30 am so there wasn't supposed to be anyone still around at all except for us. I went into the room and saw Marc's bass guitar case was open. I yelled out to Marc "Marc did you leave your bass case open?" I noticed some of our equipment close to another door that wasn't moved there by us. I ran out the door and dragged the kid back to the club realising at that point that this was the same kid that was trying to sell me equipment earlier that day. We called the police but since we weren't going to be in town anymore there wasn't much they could do. Marc and I ended up quitting the band. Soon after he went to L.A to study music and found success there while forming a few bands. Marc and I got back in touch via Facebook over thirty years later and with a renewed friendship wrote a couple of instrumentals together, one entitled 'Crossing the Caspian.'

Hans Galore (sounds like: Hands Galore)

During the Mid 1980's I worked with a

band called Hans Galore that played punk and new wave music at about 100 miles an hour. Every musician in that band played with conviction. It was high energy, great fun and I enjoyed jumping up and down behind my drum kit. Every time there was a cymbal smash that needed to be accented, I would excitedly jump up off my seat and hit the cymbal hard. For a few of the song endings, I would stand up on my drummer throne, which was actually a wooden box, do a cymbal swell and then jump back down at the end beat of the song. Physically this band was very challanging, leaving me covered in sweat from head to toe, often with sweat salt dripping into my eyes while I was playing. This was the only band that I'd ever worked with that I felt comfortable enough to be so animated like that, it was always so much fun. I learned a lot about playing with conviction with this band, which John the leader/keyboard player impressed upon me. The whole band really put on a good show, and we were well received wherever we played.

We arrived one afternoon at a bar in

cottage country, and set up our equipment. The owners were German and while me and the rest of the guys were standing on the dance floor looking at our setup, the lady owner came up to us and asked in a heavy accent "So vitch one of you is Hans?" She seemed quite disappointed that there really wasn't a Hans, it was just the name of the band. (I think it's possible that she thought we were going to be playing polkas all night). About a month later I got into a heated argument with John, the leader of the band and I quit. Even though I was asked to stay with the band after the argument was over, I was too stubborn to admit I was wrong and left the band. This pattern of arguments and fights continued and my mental health was strained.

One winter 1981ish while playing mostly around Toronto (I'm not sure what band I was playing with), I met Brenda, a young woman who was a horse groom at Woodbine Racetrack. We ended up dating for about a year. We were in love and I wrote and recorded a love song for her entitled 'You're the only one for me.' Brenda and I saw each other often even spending several nights sleeping at the racetrack in one of the cabins when it was racing season. Eventually, she felt like it wasn't going to work out and cut off all communication with me. At the same time, I had just gotten fired from the band I was in. Devastated, and in a dark place mentally, I stopped eating and sleeping, and was crying all day mostly lying in bed. At this point, I couldn't deal with any little hiccup that life would throw, which to me now was another red flag that I really needed psychiatric help. I was very fragile. I phoned my parents who could hear my distress as I sobbed uncontrollably. Dad told me he was going to come to Toronto to be with me. When he arrived, I felt so much better almost immediately. He also helped me to get my drums back from a pawn shop, staying a few more days till he was sure I was feeling better about things.

Radio Wave and Stripes

Since I needed to forget about Brenda as everything in Toronto reminded me of her, I decided to go back on the road. I just couldn't take the pain and my life felt like it was at a very low point. I joined a four-member band called Radio Wave, later taking on the name Stripes.

While playing with them in Pembroke, Ontario I dreamt one night that I was standing upstairs in a seedy hotel hallway. There was some writing on the wall, but I don't recall what it said. A man dressed in what looked like a robe came up to me and asked me if I was ready to accept God. I said "I don't know..." He looked at me with a disgusted look on his face (like, what do you mean you don't know?) and I got scared. I said, "yes I'm ready to accept God!" He told me to follow him, and I was led to a downstairs waiting room where on one side was a stairway going up and a gate with a man guarding it. In the waiting room were three chairs with two Spanish looking guys on each end. The man from the hallway told me to wait there, I sat on the middle chair. The men on either side of me were looking at playboy magazines so I also began looking with them. I looked up after a moment and noticed that the gate to the stairway was closed and the guard was gone. Becoming frightened I went up to the gate trying to find a way in. Just then, a smooth-talking man walked up to me and said, "Don't worry about it man, just go down the hallway and open the first door on your right, Don't bother to look, just walk right out there." I was suspicious and nervous so I walked up to the door and opened it while looking out first. Beyond the door was a cesspool as far as the eye could see. I walked back into the waiting room and saw that there were two port hole windows on the side of the room which looked out to the outside, but the outside was now all burnt up and barren. The two men took pickaxes and were trying to break through one of the portholes. I also took a pickaxe and started to bash away at the window. I noticed that the two men were starting to break through their window, so I started to help them.

I told this dream to our keyboard player the next day and I didn't think much more of it. After I left the band, I didn't see him for several years until one afternoon as I was taking a city bus, he got on, and we talked for a while. Before he got to his stop, he had told me that he had become a born-again Christian because of the dream I had told him that scared him so badly. He had gotten out of the music business and now was working as a dishwasher in a restaurant. I was dumbfounded and shocked at how different his life was now. Playing with Radio Wave, he had always been writing music, loved to practice new songs, and was very committed to music.

When Radio Wave changed the name of the band to Stripes, the bass player and I were the only original members remaining. We added a new guitar player, and keyboard player, with changes like this happening several times.

In the mid 1980's, Stripes and I were playing in Thunder Bay, and I had to go back to Toronto on the Sunday to move my stuff to another apartment. At this point in my life, I was moving from place to place with no solid home base. Where I had my stuff I was housesitting for that same couple of friends of mine that were again returning from Lars Germany. At first, everything went according to plan, I flew to

Toronto, finished moving and was at the airport for the return trip to Thunder Bay to rejoin the band. It was a tight schedule with our band playing again on the Monday in Hearst, a small town outside of Thunder Bay. After about an hour of delays because of issues with the planes mechanics our flight was going to be leaving, We ended up boarding the plane which seated about fifty passengers. We sat there on the tarmac for about forty-five minutes and the flight attendant came on saying there were some minor problems with the plane they were going to fix but we had to stay on the plane. An hour later, she came on again and said there were a few more problems with the plane, this time the delay was the radio wasn't working properly. She apologised. I looked out my window and saw an aircraft maintenance person standing outside shaking his head looking at the engine which was not a vote of confidence to me. I was also watching the person in the seat in front of me whose seat was broken and wouldn't go right back into position. I thought to myself this plane is a bucket of bolts and it's going to fall apart! I nervously picked up my carryon starting to walk down the aisle to get off the plane. The flight attendant stopped me at the door and said, "where are you going, we're going to be leaving in a couple of minutes?" She talked me into staying, I got back in my seat and 15 minutes later we started taxiing down the runway. The guy next to me said "Something's not right, we're not going fast enough." After about 20 seconds of getting into the air, the engines shut down and then came back on again, then almost stopped and came back on again. My heart started to race. The flight attendants were talking to the flight deck and with flushed faces started to panic, which was terrible. One of them started taking all the forward luggage and throwing it quickly into the washroom. I guess they did that in case we were going down, and they didn't want loose items to be flying around. I looked around and saw the fear in people faces with many of them crying and praying. Myself, I was numb, feeling like I was watching a movie unfold before my eyes. The pilot came on saying we had to make an emergency landing and that it had been decided we weren't going to land in Toronto after all, we were going to burn off some fuel and make a landing in Ottawa.

We were now travelling in the opposite direction of Thunder Bay and were about halfway to Ottawa when the pilot came on again and said we were going to land in Montreal instead since it had a bigger runway. The guy next to me said "Aren't you sorry you didn't get off this plane?" At that point I was nervous and was definitely feeling sorry that I didn't follow what my gut instinct was telling me. The crew were trying to keep the passengers calm by giving us some statistics that we were only cruising at about 200 miles an hour at a height of about 7000 feet if I remember correctly. Not so calming. Apparently, they were also having trouble with the nose gear and fuel pump. They gave us a lot of details, I'm not sure if it was the right thing to do. I do remember that we were very low, going really slow all the way to Montreal with the plane slowing down and speeding up and slowing down and speeding up. Once we got over Montreal, they told us to take off our shoes, put our heads down and press into to the seat in front of us. I just had to look so I peered out the window seeing flashing lights everywhere waiting for us. We came down hard, blowing a tire, but we landed safely with all the passengers clapping and letting out a huge cheer. We got off the plane, stretched and hydrated with a little bit of water and we're informed that in a couple of hours there would be another flight for us to get back to Thunder Bay. I thought to myself there was no way I was ever going to get on another plane again. Little did I know at the time, much later in my life I would meet my partner Elaine. She worked for DeHavilland Aircraft who built these planes and was the buyer of grounded aircraft parts which this aircraft would have needed. A full circle moment.

I called my Mother who had been waiting at the Thunder Bay airport at the original arrival time but since with all the delays had decided to go home to wait for additional information. I told her that I wasn't going to get back on the next plane but was going to find some other way to get back to Thunder Bay. She gently but firmly reminded me that I had to get back on the plane to play the next night. So, I did just that. I got back on the next plane which looked so new that the guy next to me said "I hope this thing has the bugs worked out of it!" It was an uneventful flight, we landed in Thunder Bay at about 5:30 AM. We had originally left Toronto at about 7:30 PM, taking so long to get to Montreal because of the slow speed we had to adhere to. I went to my parent's place for a cuppa coffee and a sandwich, then was driven straight to the bus station catching the first bus to Hearst. Having no sleep the previous night, I was laying down across the backseats of the bus the whole way. The bus was speeding up and slowing down, making a similar noise like the plane was doing. It was a nightmare, unfortunately I couldn't sleep. I arrived that afternoon in time to play the gig, so happy to see the band. They had already set up the equipment including my drums which I really appreciated. We exchanged stories about how the last 24 hours went, and I told them about the flight. Mine wasn't a happy story except for how it all ended.

Rough and Tumbling

While playing on the road with Stripes in Thunder Bay at a bar at The Sleeping Giant Motel, a lot of my extended family including my parents, some aunts, uncles, friends, and a sister-in-law and her friend were in attendance. On our first break I sat down at the table of my sister-in-law and her friend. After a while I saw out of the corner of my eye someone at another table staring at me. It felt uncomfortable so I quickly glanced over to see who it was. The guy said to me "What the fuck are you looking at?" I said "Nothing, sorry, I thought you were looking at me." He said, "Your guitar player is ok right now but will be beaten up later." I asked him what was going on and he replied, "Your guitar player made fun of a mentally challenged friend of mine." I said "I don't think Bert would do that." He said, "Are you calling me a liar?." I told him "No, I just don't think he would do that." The guy was obviously looking for a fight and was trying anything to get me to engage him in that way. He was sitting with two girls and inferred they would beat up my two lady friends. At that point, I told the girls I was sitting with we should move to another table across the room, which we did. I wasn't quite done though and being mouthy and my mental state not having any fear I walked back to the guy and said something like "This wouldn't happen in Toronto." I was wearing a skinny leather tie which he grabbed, holding me up with it and shouted, "I'll choke you with your fucking tie!" He was indeed choking me, so I had no choice but to retaliate by punching him. We grappled with each other and fell into the large speakers that were on stands near the stage causing them to fall on us. The lights in the bar came on but we continued to fight for a few more minutes. Once it was over, he threatened me by saying he was going to get an infamous local family to come finish me off. This did scare me somewhat so later after the bar closed, I took apart one of my metal cymbal stands to take to my room for protection. After I got back to my room, I called the front desk and asked them if they noticed anyone coming toward my room to call me right away. I slept uneasily that night with the metal piece under the bed just in case, thankfully, no one showed up.

My sister owned a house that she lived in and rented rooms in it to several people in the east end of Toronto. I lived there briefly around 1984. When I first moved in to Bev's house I was out of work, in a really bad place mentally, and she got me a job with Davies Demonstrating. I'd go to work several times a week demonstrating products, everything from a wet/dry shaver to the New Coke, to barbecues. Most days it was a completely different product that I'd be demonstrating. I remember having a tray of about 30 Dixie cups at a time filled with the New Coke in malls and shopping centres, having people sample them and asking them their opinion on the taste. Nobody liked it and eventually the whole "New" Coke Promotion was a huge failure, (or a success? there was a lot of talk about it in the press). They eventually pulled the product. With the wet/dry men's shaver that I was demonstrating at Eatons, Sears, and other big retailers I ended up selling about 350 of them over a six-week period near Christmas. Being the top seller, I really enjoyed demonstrating it, having a little bucket of water which I dunked the shaver into to show people that it could be used in the shower as well. The jobs with Davies entailed mostly demonstrating, but sometimes making sales were involved, which I didn't enjoy quite as much.

While I was living at Bev's house, Trevor, one of her tenants took me to see a guitar he was building at his work at Downtown Music, a guitar repair shop. It was there that I met Mike, the owner, which started a lasting friendship. Many afternoons I would stop by the shop and bring coffees for Mike and staff and shoot the breeze for about an hour. At the time, Mike had a very nice band called Bats On Skis whom I ended up playing a couple gigs with. One gig was at The Spadina Hotel which became Global Village Backpackers, the backpack hostel I would stay at years later when visiting Toronto for a month at a time.

I was starting to struggle again mentally getting more and more depressed with my self-esteem and confidence being low, most days lying-in bed rocking myself to music and not working for long periods.

Later, I ended up getting a job at a market research company calling people on the phones and met Sarah who also worked there. We started dating and several weeks later she moved in with me at my sister's house while I was still struggling mentally. At the time, sister Bev was doing many different types of jobs one of which was clowning and she had Sarah and I fill in for her for a weekend. Bev helped us out getting clowning clothes together and putting on our makeup for the job which was with a furniture manufacture that sold direct to the public. After our first weekend we were hired permanently to work four days a week for them, and Sarah and I moved into a one bedroom apartment in the west end.

We continued with the clowning job which consisted of running and dancing up and down the street wearing a sandwich board sign over our clown clothes and pointing to the direction of the company. As well, we would answer questions and hand out flyers while stopping traffic. The sign we wore said "Buy direct from the factory today" which was not quite true as they sold to the public every day. We would stand in front of the competition like The Brick, Pascals etc. and stop and direct the traffic to "our" company. We also had a system where on Dundas Street in Mississauga we'd wait until the traffic stopped at the lights, walk up to the first car and once they opened their window, hand them a flyer and continue down the line of traffic slowing the cars almost to a standstill. When the traffic resumed moving fast we would get out of the way and move back onto the sidewalk. This Dundas Street area was known for its many furniture companies. The tensions got so bad that once when we were stopping traffic outside a furniture store one of the company's managers came outside and pushed me, telling me to get out of there. That shook me up quite a bit. Several of the companies called the police on us, however, the police eventually just said there was nothing they could do as we weren't breaking any laws. Otherwise, it was a good job, paid very well (about 20 dollars an hour in the 1980's) and was great exercise.

One of the most joyful things was seeing the kid's reaction in the cars when they would see the clowns dancing on the sidewalk. My long time partner Elaine who lived in that area at the time has told me that she remembers seeing us many times running up and down the street and would always say to her kids in the backseat of the car "Wave to the clowns!" This was another time our paths had crossed. With this type of clowning job there were only a few challenges. For example, some people would throw snowballs at us, or a few overly excited children would kick our shins. Overall, it was a wonderful experience. Sarah, and I broke up at the end of a little over two years and because of my unpredictability and combative attitude we lost our job and I had sabotaged our relationship. I was very saddened by this.

I've realized now that I was suffering with mental illness in my teens and throughout my music career. I was at times violent, argumentative, and combative which hurt me a lot in my personal and professional life. In my band playing years I would quit or get fired and lay in bed for weeks, so depressed, then as inexplicably snap out of it. I wasn't diagnosed until I was thirty and I had more major symptoms of Schizophrenia which statistically usually starts in early teens. For me it was much later that full-blown schizophrenia came upon me and I stopped being able to function mentally or look after myself.

My parents helped me out financially many times, but also I would go home and work in the greenhouses from winter to spring, save a bit of money then go back to Toronto and try the music business again. I worked at the greenhouses for about six of twelve winters that I lived in Toronto. Around 1984, I wanted to take a music degree program at Humber College and asked my parents for help financially with that. They wouldn't support that idea as they didn't see music as a viable career choice. At this point, I was already into them for a lot of money. I realized later that I wouldn't have had the focus to really apply myself to the studying required to learn. I just wasn't able to learn in a structured setting at that point, my stress levels were through the roof, and I had low self-confidence. It was the right decision they made at the time, but it was hard for me to hear, since music was about the only thing that really made me feel good about myself. They've always been so supportive in every other way and I'm sure they just wanted to protect me. At this point, nobody knew including myself that I had a mental illness. Even when I did have a day job, it wouldn't last more than a few months and I'd get into an argument and quit. I would've been much better off with some stability in my life. During the four years that I worked with lounge bands and was only playing in Toronto I was mostly able to be independent of my parents help. To help relieve stress in my life every night after work around 2:00 am I would run at the track across the street from the house I was ,living in. The track was located between two schools and I usually ran about 20 laps. During the day I'd also go for a run around the east end area. With all the stuff going on in my head, all the worry, I found this very invigorating, and the runs would give me a great sense of peace inside. Unfortunately, my being ill, unreliable and argumentative got me fired so often that finally I got a bad name in the lounge circuit, and no one would hire me anymore.

For three years ending in 1987, I was living at The Hotel Isabella, a five-story hotel renting to musicians downtown. The rent was exactly $152.50 for the month for musicians. I always wondered what the 50 cents was for. It was surreal as during those years I was playing at most of the high-end show rooms and lounges at night while living in the very humble 100-year-old place that I could afford. I remember the newspaper ads for the hotel back in the day would say 'Get Dizzy at the Izzy.' Living there did have some challenges. There were no fridges in the rooms so I would keep my milk, cheese and groceries on the windowsill in the winter. As well, occasionally the radiator in the overly hot room would spew a stream of water. The Izzy had its own haunted house stories with young, tall and lean Russell, one of the employees telling us of when he was in the basement one evening an empty beer case went whizzing by his head. Russel would often walk around the main floor and for a laugh would hit the counter with a baseball bat while yelling Bam! (The bat normally residing behind the front desk for the staff's protection).

I lived on the 2nd floor of the six-floor building and some of my neighbors were Michael, a very talented blues harp player/singer and Ben and Leanne, a couple, Ben being an amazing drummer and Leanne, a wonderful person and talented musician. The night manager and bartender was a big friendly guy but also tough as nails. Some of the staff and I had a fun rivalry going with the score on the Donkey Kong game. The night manager was usually the high score winner and would post messages on the game challenging anyone to beat his score which I proudly did but not really that often.

There were four or five bars at the hotel, three of them having entertainment which over the years I played in many times. As well, there was a great jam every weekend in the bar downstairs where many local musicians like me would sit in and play. I remember seeing Peter Tork from The Monkees play a show down there. It was a wonderful way to meet many great musicians that I never would have otherwise, and it was actually a very good time in my life for personal growth. One day while I was practicing my singing in my room and I'd stop, I could hear laughing in the room next to mine. A few days later Michael told me I didn't need to practice and that I could sing already. I guess he got tired of hearing me sing the song 'Can't Hurry Love' over and over and over again. Through living at the hotel, I met Wally, an excellent, solid drummer whom I bumped into several years ago after not talking to him for about 40 years. He didnt remember me at first till I told him about my living on the second floor of the Izzy. I look completely different now, back in the day having shoulder length dark hair and weighing 135 pounds.

C.J Feeney, one of the members of the 60's Blues band 'The Sparrows' was a great musician and singer who had a unique style of standing while having his guitar strap and guitar very low with slightly bent legs, playing with his thumb down on the fretboard. When I had the honour to get to know him, he was a bartender in the back bar on the main floor and would perform there often. Unfortunately, we all had to move out of the hotel when the building was sold and renovated into a more high-end establishment. I have great memories from that time even though my family wondered why I was living in such a dive. Personally, I appreciated the great camaraderie and laid-back atmosphere of the hotel and I felt like I was paying my dues while learning how to be a better human being and drummer.

Cherrill Rae

One of the last bands I worked with in Toronto was with Cherrill Rae, whom I idolised as a younger musician. Her original act called The Raes had a number of hits on the radio which spawned a successful TV series under that name. Unfortunately, after working with her for several months, I wasn't looking after my drum equipment, it was falling apart including cymbals with big pieces out of them and I was also getting into arguments with the bass player. One night I did a drum fill where I lost my focus leaving the band fall apart with everyone including our professional dancers stopping the show and looking at me. A few weeks later we were playing at Pier 4, a beautiful harbor nightclub that I often played at with several bands in Toronto when Cherrill took me aside and gave me my two week's notice which was really bad timing as I had only just bought new drums partially on credit but hadn't picked them up yet. I was not functioning very well at all and I know that she did the right thing by letting me go. My caliber of playing at that time was nowhere near her level.

Vince Fraser

I was out of work and was shopping at Long and McQuade's (a local music store) one day when one of the drums salesmen said to me "Keith, this guy needs a drummer, are you available?" This guy (Vince) had me sit at a drum kit right there in the showroom to see if I could play Soca, a West Indian rhythm which he demonstrated, I played it, he told me he thought I played it with feeling, and I got the job. It was a Caribbean music band, and we were playing for a couple weeks at Lions head, on a beautiful resort near Owen Sound. Before leaving Toronto, we had to pick up Pablo who was going to play bass with us. We arrived at Pablo's apartment building and Vince went in and buzzed telling him we were there. We waited and waited but Pablo didn't come out of the building. Vince went in several more times and buzzed, at this point having waited about an hour. Vince finally went upstairs to find Pablo wallpapering his Livingroom, oblivious that we were possibly going to get to the gig late. He took another half hour or so, finished the job and came downstairs with his equipment. I was meeting everyone in the band as they got in the van. We also had 'Tunka' with us who as a part of the show would walk on broken wine and beer bottles with his bare feet without getting even a scratch, later performing the limbo while dancing underneath very low sticks. As well, he would ask the crowd to go outside with him where he would take big swigs of gasoline and quickly spew out the gas from his mouth while lighting it with a torch, the flames billowing ten to fifteen feet into the air. The crowd would applaud and cheer during his flame act, I'm sure that most of them had never before seen anything quite like it in person. I often wonder where Tunka and other musicians I worked with are now. Some I've been able to reconnect with.

On the way back from that job, we were travelling down the highway when a man and woman on a motorcycle pulled out in front of us and slowed down stopping sideways, blocking us from driving any further. Still on the bike, the guy rolled up to Vince's window who was driving and said that we had cut them off and started to argue with Vince. He then asked me what I was doing in this car with a bunch of (*racial slurs). I said, "They're my friends." He went to pull something out from behind him but his girlfriend who was riding on the back of the motorcycle with him shouted "No!" He pulled his hand back and took off on his bike leaving us all a little shaken.

I worked with 26 bands over 12 years in Toronto, 1976 to 88. "I couldn't keep a job" is a little joke I used to make but it was mostly true. Another joke I liked using during my band days was saying to the band leader that if I was going to leave the band, "I'd give notice." Then saying, it would be in the form of a note left on the drumless stage saying, "as you've probably noticed I've left the band." There were only certain people I'd use that little joke with. The styles of bands I worked with ranged from soca, reggae and calypso to lounge bands playing dinner music to disco, funk, rock 'n' roll, rhythm and blues and country. Some of the show bands I worked with we had matching stage clothes and costume changes and put on a show which sometimes included a lot of stage lighting and pyrotechnics. At the time, I was smoking two large packs a day and drinking way too much. I was definitely not well and not always eating properly or sleeping much.

I've never driven in Toronto or on the road with bands that I worked with. Not having a vehicle, I had to rely on one of the band members to move my drums around in their van or car, or sometimes taking cabs or planes wherever I needed to go.

With one in-town band, I forgot that we were doing a showcase for agents to get bookings and didn't show up for it. The band ended up using a drummer from one of the other bands for the audition. A total embarrassment for myself and very unprofessional of me. With that band I also was late leaving my teaching drums job in Mississauga one night, which made me over an hour late for our gig at a hotel by the airport. The buses were not running on time and the leader of the band had to leave the club and pick me up at a bus stop. I was soon fired and blamed them, but really, they were totally in the right to let me go, I was not dependable at that time in my life. I was always feeling lost and was totally disorganised.

Over my life I've had many spiritual topic dreams as well as dreams about aliens. This is one I'd like to share that I had around 1986. I dreamt that I was walking down a hill by my old public school when I saw a disc shaped spacecraft of some kind laying at the bottom of the hill. Two human looking beings approached me and took me on board. As we began moving, I noticed a video monitor showing what appeared to be the Earth on it. We got further away from the Earth, it got smaller and smaller in the monitor. Just before it disappeared completely, I saw the Earth explode. It was gone. I asked one of the men what it was, and he said, "It's your home." I started to cry and started begging for another chance. Just then he turned to the other man and winked.

One winter afternoon in Toronto I was at a local indoor mall and spotted a homeless man laying down on a bench. The man wasn't bothering anyone but was being thrown out by security. I asked the security guard why he was hassling the man and he said, "I'm just doing my job!" Trying to help the homeless man, I gently took him by the hand to the mall coffee shop and gave the barista ten dollars enabling him to stay out of the cold as long for as he wanted to that day. Upon leaving the coffee shop, sadness came upon me for the injustices of the world. In my heart I sombrely asked God "Why?" At that moment, I felt like I was physically being drawn in the direction of a record shop, stopping at one of the record bins. In front of me was my answer, it was an album by the band Earth, Wind, and Fire entitled "That's The Way Of The World."

A COMPLETE MENTAL BREAKDOWN

In 1988, just before my break down, I was living at a house with Tina and Berk. Tina was a woman I had met a few years earlier at the By The Way Cafe a favorite spot of mine, and we dated briefly later becoming good friends. While at the house my last full-time job was looking after tropical plants in office towers in Toronto. I was getting more and more undependable and not showing up for all my contracted offices instead going to a park during the day, listening to the live bands that were playing. Finally, I just up and quit.

This was the time of my spiritual journey during which I read a lot of books about spirituality. I remember feeling so great and alive that at one point when I was living with Tina and Berk I was dancing by myself in our living room to music and everything felt so free. From my spiritual book readings, I figured that it might be a good idea to start fasting for a couple of weeks drinking and eating very little. I thought I was having a serious religious experience. During my fasting, I took on a job as a waiter at The By The Way Cafe. At this point I had already stopped eating for about a week and was not shaving anymore.

On my very first day working there, I was very paranoid feeling consumed with fear, that my life was in danger and was out of control. I was sure in my mind that there was some great conspiracy and I could be murdered at any time. The owner of the restaurant asked me to go downstairs to pick up some falafel mix from a Tupperware bin that was in a room. Once downstairs, I saw a sign on the bins lid that said, "Keep closed." Confused, I thought there was no way I was going to open that up with the sign telling me not to. (This to me shows how my breakdown was skewing my thinking process). I went back upstairs and told the owner that the sign said 'keep closed'. At the end of the day he told me it wasn't going to work out, kindly paid me for the day, and I left.

I started walking on the streets in bare feet for several weeks stepping on broken glass and stones on purpose thinking it was a very spiritual thing to do. I needed to feel pain. I developed major callouses on the bottoms of my feet. I walked to the Eaton centre downtown noticing that many people in the area were wearing sunglasses. I thought they were angels, and that the sunglasses were to hide their pure looking eyes, keeping their identities secret. I stood in front and started to speak loudly to anyone passing by that would listen saying, "The Roman Catholic Church controls billions of dollars of assets while many people in the world are starving!" An old man sitting on a bench, whom I thought was the Devil, stood up, came up to me and yelled "I'm Roman Catholic! what are you saying about the church?" I kept talking and repeating what I was saying to which he said "You're flogging a dead horse! Stop it!" and started pushing me around. At that point, I remembered something from the Bible about telling the devil to get behind you, so I said, "Get behind me Satan!" and the man did, pushing me to the ground several times telling me to stop what I was saying. A young man who had sunglasses on that I also thought was an angel was very kind, and he got between the two of us. He stopped the old man (who had what appeared to be dirty magazines stuck down the front of his pants) from pushing me around telling him to leave me alone and to pull his pants up. I asked the kind man if I could see his eyes and he lifted his sunglasses. I cried thinking that I had just seen an angel's eyes and said to him "They're beautiful!" He just smiled. After a few more minutes I stopped my preaching, the old man left, and then so did I, walking several miles uptown to a movie theatre where I had heard on the news *The Last Temptation of Christ*, a very controversial movie, was playing. When I arrived, in front of the theatre an older priest was leading his congregation around in circles in support of their Savior by protesting the movie. I'm sure they were thinking they were doing a good thing, but I started spouting off about the church again yelling things like "Oh hypocrites!" A young woman who was with the congregation said to me "Leave them alone they're old people" I felt really bad, so I left and went to a nearby street corner, continuing to speak my piece when another young woman hearing me came by and handed me a bouquet of beautiful flowers. That random act of kindness touched me deeply.

My mind was not focused and was all over the place with fear and conflicting ideas. I decided I should walk across the United States barefoot for charity. That night, I went to the Toronto bus station randomly choosing to get a ticket for a bus leaving for Cincinnati, Ohio in the next hour which sounded perfect to me. I bought a one-way ticket which I didn't realise I needed a return one. Once we got to the border, they had us all get out of the bus. The U.S Border officer asked me a bunch of questions and looked through my bag which had only a bible, a few pairs of socks and a few other light clothes. He was not impressed, telling me he wasn't going to let me into the U.S. I had to wait a few hours for a return bus to Toronto and once arriving went back home to the house in Toronto that I lived at with Tina and Berk.

Undaunted, the next day I took a day bus to the border again but this time trying to get across to Buffalo New York. I got a return ticket and arrived several hours later. We all got off the bus and the Border Officer could see on his computer that I had been turned away trying to go to Cincinnati the night before. I got in a huge argument with him and I said the U.S needs us more than we need them. He didn't like that comment and asked what they needed Canada for. I continued to shoot off my big mouth and said, "For drinking water once yours is all polluted." He was infuriated and with that comment, took me outside where he threatened me saying, "If you ever come back to this border you'll leave in an ambulance." I returned to Toronto and the house once again.

A few days later, I started to get more paranoid and was hearing and seeing things. Things people were saying seemed directed at me even as they were just passing me on the street. I remember being so confused at home and throwing a drum, breaking my bedroom window. I also let Tina's pet bird go free. I felt bad about the whole thing, and I blamed it on someone breaking into the house which of course was not true. My roommates didn't question what I was saying, but years later I told them the truth.

I was running out of money at this time and decided to downsize all my possesions including my drums taking a taxi with all my equipment way up Yonge Street to a drum shop. I ended up gettng about 500 dollars in the form of a cheque but I also needed some cash as I didn't have any money to pay for the cab that brought me there. Luckily the drum shop obliged and covered my taxi cost.

One night I was watching my T.V and was hearing things on T.V I thought were directed at me. I picked it up while it was on and smashed it on the floor completely breaking it. Later that night, I was hearing people screaming my name on the street when I was trying to sleep, and I saw a scorpion on the floor in my room which went and hid under a chair. It looked so real, but even with the fear, the exhaustion took over. I just lay down to rest.

After not sleeping at all for days, one day I noticed there were many butterflies around the bush in front of our house which looked so beautiful. The next day there were many bees in that same spot. I started clapping the bees in my hands killing them all, oddly enough not getting stung once. I had enough and walked out the door that day never going back, ending up on the streets. I was so disappointed years later when I realised the people I was living with at the time, did not even make an attempt to find me or find out what happened to me after I disappeared from the house one day leaving all my belongings there. Thinking back to that time, I'm pretty sure I was probably scaring everybody with my unpredictability. Tina did have my parents phone number but never called them nor sent my personal things including a pine bed, cassette tapes of bands and band photos and memorabilia. Apparently, she gave my belongings to the actual owner of that house who did hang on to my things for years but threw it all out by the time I was well enough to inquire about it.

One night on the street not having eaten anything for a long period of time or drinking hardly any water my body was feeling numb. I was pinching myself and couldn't feel anything. As I walked by a brick building, I hit it as hard as I could with my fist to see if I would feel anything, I didn't…. Nothing. A little while later I felt an energy in my legs, and I started to run down the street so fast that I was almost falling forward. I ran by some guy on the street who yelled "Fuck off" at me. I walked the streets for several days, maybe weeks.

I remember one day outside at City Hall running around laughing and trying to give passerby's a $20-dollar bill. Finally, a young teenage girl took it, causing me to run away hysterically laughing thinking that my job was done. I somehow ended up camping out on the steps of Much Music on Queen Street downtown. When I first got there, I was overcome with emotion about what was going on in my mind and got down on my hands and knees and was sobbing uncontrollably. A passerby came by and put his arm over my back and said, "Are you OK, are you OK?" I can't remember what I said but I was very touched by his act of kindness. I stayed in front of the building for two or three days chain smoking. At one point somebody from Much Music came out and told me that they didn't mind me staying there, but just keep the area clean of cigarette butts and to not make a mess. A passerby said to me, "Give into it!" I said to him "I'm nothing" feeling that I wasn't even worthy of life and he said, "You should have a higher opinion of yourself." One night the police came by, and I was under my blanket too afraid to look out. They were grabbing at the blanket trying to see who was under it and were kicking at my shins with their hard boots which really hurt. They told me to move on, so I did.

Walking around downtown another day, I saw three jet planes scream past. In my mind, thinking they were angels not airplanes. I now realize that it was around the time of the Canadian National Exhibition, and they were probably from the airshow. Around the same time, I also remember going into a variety store and asking the owner if I could eat some green beans that he had outside by the front display that had spilled to the ground. He said of course and I picked them up eating a small handful. Later, I walked to a park and lay on the ground thinking I could hear a water pump pumping under me. I had no idea what was happening to me as my whole world had been flipped upside down. My new "reality" did not make any sense to me.

I remember trying to get warm one time during the day and sitting inside in the doorway of a building, security coming and kicking me out. It was a terrible feeling. That and so many other ways where I was treated badly has made me gentler and have more empathy toward people that are homeless and those suffering from mental illness. At first, when I'd left the house, I had a winter jacket on but after a few days I didn't trust it as it smelled strange to me and left it on a street corner. I had a little bit of money so after a few very chilly nights I bought a blanket. It was now fall, and was quite chilly in Toronto at night.

Having enough of being out of doors on cold nights, I ended up in a hostel downtown. When I first arrived, I was warned by another homeless person to keep my runners under my pillow at night so no one could steal them. That night there was a guy in a bed next to me that had gotten up to go do something in the next room. I saw he had a bag by his bed and in my mind I thought there might be something magical in the bag that I needed for the mission my mind was telling me I was on. I wasn't sure what it was, but I needed to get into that bag. I carefully started looking through it. There was a peanut butter sandwich in there as well as a bunch of other things. He returned, saw what I was doing, and of course was quite upset with me. Staff moved me to another room away from him. The next night I tried to get into the same hostel, but they turned me away most likely because I went through that guy's possessions.

Many negative thoughts about dying and getting murdered were going around in my head during this time frame. At first, late one night I walked along the highway 401 in Toronto with lanes of eighteen wheelers and many other types of vehicles screaming fast by me. It was very dangerous although at the time I didn't feel any danger. To try and calm my thoughts, a few days or so later I started walking west from downtown all the way to Oakville, about 24 miles. It took hours and hours basically the whole day and night.

On the way, when I got to Mississauga, I noticed the sidewalks had little dried berries in many varieties all over with not a tree or bush in sight. At one point on my way I went to a farm where they were selling fruit and vegetables and asked if I could have something to eat, they just said no. So very hungry, I continued on. Once I got to Oakville, I decided to start making my way back to Toronto but was so tired that what I really needed was rest. It was dark and in the wee hours, so I laid down on the sidewalk of all places because I thought it was safer. What seemed like a few minutes after laying there I heard sirens and saw lights flashing. Someone had called an ambulance thinking that I was hurt or had died right on the sidewalk. The police arrived, took my ID, looked at it and told me to go back to Toronto since it was another division, and the other division would have to deal with me. I remember on my way back that day just walking and walking, still in bare feet and finding side roads to walk down and not knowing where I was going.

Continuing on my way back to Toronto, I arrived back in Mississauga during the night. I looked on the opposite side of the street and much to my amazement I saw the silhouettes of many pyramids. I had no idea where I was anymore. It started pouring rain and I was soaked to the skin and cold so I asked at a restaurant if I could come in, rest and get dry to which they agreed. They were very kind. I was about to leave at one point, and the owner said, "just stay for a while longer, take it easy!" Once again, I was very touched by that act of kindness; I'm sure by looking at my unshaven face and wild uncombed hair he knew I was in trouble mentally. Later, I walked by a little factory which was making Pita bread. There was a door open off the street and I looked in and I asked the person who looked like he might be the owner if I could have a pita as I was very hungry. Obviously irritated he asked, "Why should I do that for you nobody's ever done anything for me?" That made me feel like the lowest of the low, but he gave me a pita anyway which I ended up not eating as I was afraid of it.

I went into a grocery store and asked the owner if there was anything I could do to make some money so I'd be able to buy a little bit of food to eat. He said they had no job for me but took me to the back room where there was a little bushel basket of apples and gave it to me. When I got back on the street, I ate one or two of the apples which were Macintosh. They tasted so very sweet, and I couldn't eat any more, leaving the rest by the side of the road. I didn't like 'them' apples. I kept walking, finally making my way to the outer west end of Toronto.

I've never told employers about my illness, as I always assumed they wouldn't take a chance on hiring me. So, in the past I would alter my work history slightly when applying to account for the lost years in hospital and healing. Any of the people I have worked for (after I became well) will tell you that I am a conscientious and reliable worker, on time always and work hard. I've never had any complaints from bosses or anyone.

Trying to deal with many conflicting thoughts of being tortured and murdered, I somehow thought that to get away I should hitchhike south to Windsor Ontario, about five hours away. I went into a truck stop and asked the patrons there if anyone was going south. A truck driver spoke up and offered me a ride. Once in Windsor, I slept outside for a couple of nights on benches, still not eating or drinking. One night the police stopped by in a patrol car and asked me what I was doing, telling me to go to a hostel. I told them I was too afraid do that.

In the afternoon of the next day, I went into a corner store and was so paranoid but was starving for something to eat. I was about to purchase a chocolate bar but kept checking and rechecking the ingredients to make sure that it wasn't something that would kill me. I could see the owner was watching me the whole time probably trying to figure out what I was doing. I bought the bar, stepped out of the store and ate it. Still paranoid, and thinking I had just eaten poison, I went into the parking lot, crouched down on my hands and knees and put my fingers down my throat making myself sick. The store owner came out and shouted, "What are you doing? don't ever come back here again!" Deciding to go back to Toronto, that night I ended up hitchhiking back with another truck driver, helping him deliver some packages on the way. The heavy metal music he was playing in the truck seemed evil to me and I was nervous and wary of him. We arrived near Toronto the next morning and he was letting me off on a ramp to the highway saying he was bypassing the city. I was feeble and weak at this point about three weeks into a fast without much water and as I got out of the truck and he left, I heard a horn and was nearly hit by a car.

I got to a payphone and called my parents telling them that I was not well, and that I wanted to come home to Thunder Bay. They sent me a plane ticket which I picked up at the airport, walking to get there. I still had my passport at this time but had thrown away my wallet with all my other ID. Arriving in Thunder Bay with only the clothes on my back, I was very skinny since I hadn't been eating for quite a while. When Dad saw me, he said "Jesus!" (Rob told me that is who Dad thought I looked like when he saw me with the long hair and beard). At first, for several days, I was still scared and confused and had trouble getting my words out so afraid to say anything that could result in my being murdered by friends, by family, anyone. I was also still smoking two packs a day and every time I lit a cigarette, I thought it would result in my being murdered for this sin. Even with these terrifying, convinced thoughts of imminent death it still took me several months to quit smoking which gave me a lot of empathy for people who are trying to quit smoking as to how really hard it is. I would find out later that my parents were worried, and my mother, scared about how out of it I was hid all the sharp knives not giving me access to them. I'm sure they didn't have any idea what I was capable of in that state. However, I was sure of one thing, I wasn't capable of harming anybody except myself. I started eating again with the love and gentle prodding of my parents and got back to working at the greenhouses.

In the spring of 1989 after seeming to be well for a while I decided I wanted to go to Israel and work on a Kibbutz which is a commune and there are over 300 of them in Israel. In my mid-twenties while I was living with Sarah whom I used to clown with, her brother had come back from Israel and had worked on a Kibbutz telling many interesting stories about life on one. I always thought over the years that it sounded like a great way to live. I was given some books about Israel from a Doctor friend of Dad's who lived in

Thunder Bay. I did quite a bit of research, of course it was 1989, there was no Internet or online, so it was all through reading books or hearing stories from other people. I saw that I was able to apply to volunteer once I arrived in Israel. I made all the arrangements, purchased my plane ticket, taking El AL, the Israeli airline to get there. I had to go through heavy security in the Toronto Airport to go to Israel. They took my bag to a table where they looked at the contents carefully and took the batteries out of my clock. They took a long look at my antipsychotic medication but decided to let me travel. I finally made it through security and got on the plane.

During the last part of the flight, I was amazed that most of the men went to the back of the plane and were doing prayers while bobbing their upper body up and down like you would see at The Wailing Wall in Israel. I was thinking, Is this safe with all that weight in the tail end? It was fine and we arrived at the international airport in Lod, about 20 kilometers from Tel Aviv. I got a cab to Tel Aviv and upon arriving walked around a bit enjoying a beautiful hot day in early spring. At that point I had gone off my meds for about a week and a half or two weeks without my parents knowing. I had actually already started feeling unwell a week or so before leaving Thunder Bay. Once in Israel it immediately escalated to off tastes and strong odors.

As I was lying in bed in my hotel room just looking at the ceiling, I noticed a very strong odd smell wafting in from the open window. I closed the window and was trying to decide what to do, so frightened I couldn't even go outside anymore that evening. I made the decision to leave after that first night and got myself back to the airport. Of course, being very security orientated they were extremely interested to know why, after one day, I was going back to Canada when I had a ticket booked for three months. I explained to them that I was having mental difficulty. They searched me thoroughly, went over my body with a metal detector and after about an hour of interrogation decided they would let me go back.

I got a ticket for the first plane leaving the following day, but it was going via Germany as there were no direct flights that day back to Toronto. I spent the night in the airport and headed to Frankfurt the next morning. When I arrived in Frankfurt I started having an episode, was very paranoid and resolved to get off the plane and not continue to Toronto. The problem was we were already taxiing down the runway ready to takeoff. I stopped the flight attendant as she walked by and told her I needed to get off the plane, that I was having a medical issue. They turned around going back to the terminal which I'm sure a lot of passengers weren't happy about, and I got off the plane. I wandered around the airport for the whole evening very paranoid not knowing what to do. I bought a little bit of cheese and a bun which I did not eat.

The next day I took a taxi to downtown Frankfurt by the train station and walked around the streets for the whole day back-and-forth trying to calm myself, scared out of my wits. It was starting to get dark and at that point, I had thought the day was never going to end and felt that somehow several weeks had gone by. I went back downtown and got a hotel room by the train station. The hotel smelled funny to me and so did the room, I was having all kinds of scared negative thoughts. I went down to the front desk and asked for my money back saying I couldn't stay there. The owner was none too pleased. Going outside I wandered around for about another hour and decided I did want to stay in the hotel. I went back in and told the owner I wanted to stay after all. He refused to let me stay, so I went back out into the night.

Time was warped for me; I had no concept of what day or time it was. I would find out later on, psychiatrists used knowing date, time and place as questions to assess someone's mental state before admission to hospital. For a while I walked all over Frankfurt conscious of smelling strong strange things in the air making me change direction and walk in the opposite direction of the smell only to be turned around again many times running from the odors. I ended up at bar downtown and stood in front for a little while too afraid to go in. A young woman came out eventually and asked me why I was standing there. I really didn't say much to her, I didn't know how to answer. I just moved on. I took several taxis all over the place back to the airport twice or more but each time leaving, getting another cab and going downtown. I arrived in the outskirts of the city at a hotel recommended by a cab driver, got out but was too afraid to go in. Hailing another cab, I finally went back downtown. That evening I continued to pace back-and-forth in and out of the train station for hours on end, finally collapsing in front of it. Someone called an ambulance; I was semi-conscious at the time, and they put some smelling salts under my nose to bring me around. This made me choke. They put me in the ambulance but while travelling toward the hospital I tried to get the door of the moving vehicle open to jump out. The attendant fought with me keeping me down and told me that he was stronger than I was, and he was, keeping his arm on my throat till we got to the hospital.

They took me to a psychiatric hospital where they restrained me tying my hands and feet to a bed in the ward hallway. That night, indignant, I was calling out to them to free my hands and feet. An orderly released one hand and one foot, leaving me again. I wasn't happy with that, so I continued yelling and defiantly tried to push the bed up and down the hall along the side. One of the orderlies came up to me sticking a needle into in my butt cheek, and I was knocked out like a light. The next morning, upon waking I opened my eyes to find two professional looking men at my bedside. I would later find out it was a judge and a lawyer who we're going to decide if I needed to continue to be detained in the hospital.

Since I couldn't talk from the medication, they had given me the evening before, of course they decided that I was unfit to leave. Eventually that day they took the straps off my hands and feet. Feeling so afraid of my situation I took off running as fast as I could, full force right into the locked main door trying to get out, where I collapsed on the floor. (I thought I could pass right through the door like a ghost). They helped me back to bed in the main hall and told me to just lie there and relax, which I did. One of the questions the Doctor asked me was if I had taken "some kind of drug." He was obviously trying to find out if I had a bad reaction, since I wasn't saying much, eventually figuring that I had a form of psychosis.

After a few days I was set up with a bed in one of the side rooms, sharing the room with two other patients. Because of my mental state all I could do was lay in bed all day. At first, even after being offered the bottled water which everyone else was drinking, I was only drinking the tap water. The water was just not tasting normal to me. One of the non-English speaking orderlies motioned to me to come to the sink. He pointed at the sink tap and made a grimace and then pointed to a bottle of water and put his arm up to show a muscle. So, I got the message, the sink water was polluted, and bottled water was safe. I started drinking the bottled water.

One night one of my roommates was talking loudly with someone else in our room as I was trying to sleep. I asked him to go talk outside of the room to which he responded, "Do you want something here?" while putting his fist up to his face. I said, "You're going to hit me for nothing?" He replied, "Because, I am nothing!" I felt bad that he really believed he was unworthy and nothing, very similar to what I said and believed in Toronto. I didn't have much communication with the other twenty or so patients on the ward as they were all speaking German and I was feeling somewhat intimidated and lost. After several days, I was allowed to go down the stairs at the back of the ward to what they called the garden which had a little patch of grass, a park bench and a few little birds landing in and out. It was a very humble garden with a high barbwire fence, but I was grateful to at least see some sunshine.

By this time, Dr. Nispel, the very kind psychiatrist who was seeing me told me that the hospital had contacted the Canadian Consulate who in turn got in touch with my parents. My Dad had no choice but to come to Germany to pick me up and bring me back to Canada. I had already been in hospital for ten days, had been evaluated, and they were obliged to release me to the care of my father. The day my Dad arrived, we got a hotel room for the night. When we arrived at the airport the next morning I was still feeling unwell from the medication I was prescribed. We told the staff at the airport that I was very sick and they agreed to let me into the Pilot's lounge where I could lay down. They put Dad and I on a shuttle trolly and took us through the airport with the lady driving it intermittently saying *Achtung!* to get everyone's attention that we were coming through. Once in the lounge one of the flight attendants asked me what was wrong with me, and I just said, "I don't want to talk about it" as it really was none of her business. I was so ill, I couldn't walk around, the only thing I could do was lay down on a bench in a fetal position and try and keep my thoughts positive.

The next day after we got back to Thunder Bay, I went to see a psychiatrist. I told him which medication I was on and that's when he told me it was not available in North America or used here. This doctor did not prescribe any medication at first and I went home to my parents where I continued to work at the greenhouses for a while. Since I was lying in bed most of the day, a major saving grace for me along with my parents during that time period was our dog, a big black female standard poodle. She would come downstairs as soon as my parents would go out for a bit and either lay in the bed with me or crawl under until they came home. I found that to be so very comforting.

In September of 1989, I had been stable for a while, but my parents had noticed that I was staring while not focussing on anything in particular. I also was not really watching the TV anymore. I had stopped taking my meds, stopped eating, showering and sleeping, and was keeping the light on all night in fear.

One morning, I was out of my mind with fear walking through the greenhouses. I was scared out of my wits and foaming at the mouth. I looked at a power panel thinking it had flames billowing out of it. The plants were giving off an odd, deep, pungent odor and everything looked and felt very dark and scary. Once Dad realised I was in a worse condition than in the previous days, he told me he should take me to the hospital, so I agreed to go.

It was the hospital I was born in, this time seeing a psychiatrist who asked a bunch of questions I was too afraid to answer. I tried to leave the room to get away, but Dad stood in my way at the door. I tried to get past him, but he grabbed me by the hair leaving him with a handful as I broke away. The psychiatrist said "no, no, let him leave!" I went outside and started wandering around not knowing what to do, feeling like I was someone else, not the musician I had been for years, that all seemed so far away now. The General Hospital called the police who arrived in minutes and took me to the Psychiatric Hospital, but since

I didn't recognize the building and didn't know where I was, I thought I had gone to another dimension and was no longer in this world. That was my first hospital admission in Thunder Bay.

At first, during my first admission at that Hospital, I was getting about eight or ten visits a day from relatives which I just couldn't handle; I couldn't get the energy up to face anybody and was too afraid to answer any of their questions. To me, even answering how I was doing felt like a loaded question with the sentences having double meanings and inuendo. I had to tell Mom and Dad to tell them all not to come, I really needed peace and time to heal right then. Some of them would still come at times during future hospital stays but not as often. Looking back, I do appreciate the thoughtfulness and caring of their visits.

Most days I wouldn't want to see anybody, but there were also other times in later admissions where Mom would come, and I told the staff I didn't want to see her. She would advise them to tell me again that his mother is there to see him, and I would finally get up and go see her. Dad would visit often, with visits from anyone taking place on the ward in a small but quiet side room.

While Dad was visiting me one day a patient that had just been admitted was put in a side room and was laying on the floor in a strait jacket yelling and kicking away at the door making a lot of noise. (The door had a round window in it so patients could be observed). The next day Dad came back to visit and was having a nice conversation with a patient in the hallway. After the patient went elsewhere Dad asked me who he was. I told him he was the same guy who was kicking at the door and making all the noise yesterday. My Dad couldn't believe it. This is a good example of how dramatic the change in behaviours can be when someone that is out of control is put on medication. That patient and I became good friends and are still in touch often.

December 1989

After several weeks on the medication

(Haldol) I was released to the care of my parents to stay at their home. Only a week or two after being released from Hospital I went off my medication once again and was not eating, showering or sleeping. My parents called the psychiatrist who I had been seeing and he came to my parents' home. He asked me a few questions and called the police when it was evident that my thinking was seriously impaired, and I'd refused medication even though he several times had asked me to take it. The police came and returned me to Hospital.

In my second hospital admission I refused meds and food. I was spending days in bed, most of the time not able to get up, so depressed and paranoid that all I could do was lay in a ball. After a couple weeks I was brought before the Ontario Review Board with The Patient Advocate defending me. The internet explains what a review board consists of:

"The ORB is comprised of a five-person panel. The chair is a retired judge or senior lawyer, and members include at least one psychiatrist, one lawyer, one individual licensed to practice either psychology or medicine and one lay person."

My Dad was present at these review board to testify that I wasn't able to make my own decisions. The Patient Advocate argued on my behalf. This was very hard for Dad each time. The Board had to decide whether I was fit to make my own decisions or not. The criteria for them to keep me in hospital is if I'm a danger to someone else or a danger to myself. It was never that I was a danger to someone else, but only to myself by staying off meds and starving myself because of fear. The actual third criteria is serious impairment to self which is what they admitted me and held me with every time.

When I was brought into the room with the review board for the first time I waited until everybody arrived, then said jokingly "I guess you're wondering why I brought you all here?" (they all laughed at that). I agreed that I'd start eating again and I wouldn't try to leave the hospital, staying, instead of trying to get my freedom back.

So far, feeling imprisoned, I had been refusing medication. After the review board hearing I continued to go downhill. Sometimes I would try to eat, but because the food tasted and smelled extremely off to me, I would immediately run to the bathroom and make myself sick by putting my fingers down my throat. The taste and the foul smells I was experiencing made me think that the food was evil and that I was possibly being poisoned. After about six weeks of not taking medication, not having eaten anything and drinking little water I was near death and down to under 100 pounds having been about 140 pounds when I was admitted.

Several times every day the staff were trying to get me to eat. I could hear the TV in the lunchroom playing music every day, all day. Often times, it was heavy metal music or other music that someone was putting on which I was finding hidden meanings in. Sometimes I would gather my strength, get up to shut the TV off or change the channel, but the music would be turned back on again most likely by a patient. I was often hearing voices say the words "oh! dead!" and when I would think a hopeful thought a voice would say, "Hope" meaning to me I shouldn't be hoping as there was no hope for me.

One afternoon while lying in bed I was going over and over in my head the very old song "Mares eat oats and does eat oats and little lambs eat ivy, a kid will eat ivy too, wouldn't you?" When I got to the part "a kid will eat ivy too," I heard Joan Rivers say on the TV "Not my kids!" which kind of made me laugh to myself. One night, I was retching in bed and throwing up only bile, not getting out of bed to do so. I could hear a nurse down the hall asking another "who is retching?" Within a day or two I had to go through the review board but this time, they decided it was an emergency and therefore wouldn't violate my rights to be put on medications. They hoped that I would start eating again. The staff brought me back to my room, offering me meds, again asking me if I would take them, I refused. They told me what would happen if I refused, and I refused again. Two male nurses came in, grabbed me and put me in a side room on a bed. They took down my trousers, held me down and stuck a needle with Haldol in my butt cheek. I was so humiliated, but they were trying to save my life. I pleaded in my weakened state "No! Don't!" I was too weak to fight them but also so afraid to die.

After a little while they came back, carried me to the bathroom, put me into the tub and bathed me. Soon after that, I was put into some pyjamas, ending up in a locked room with a bed for observation. I would understand later that this was what I needed at the time and it was all in my best interest. Although feeling defeated there was a slight bit of relief that the decision to take medication was made for me. The nurses didn't give me anything to stop the side effects of the Haldol which they normally do so after about a couple hours my whole mouth couldn't close, and it was opening wider and wider and wider with my jaw locked. I was in a lot of pain which they finally saw and gave me some meds to stop that from continuing.

Several times Dad fought for me at the

review board when I was too sick to make rational decisions. If not for him and the efforts of the nursing staff, I'm sure now that I would have died from starvation. Over a four-year period, I would have nine hospital admissions (ten, counting Germany) This was only the second one, but the one I remember the most about. The experiences I mention are very similar for most of my admissions.

I was in and out of hospital so many times, going in front of the review board each time that it became a revolving door. The decisions became quicker and quicker as it just became more and more apparent that I couldn't look after myself and I wasn't rational. The recurring pattern became; my parents would tell me to go to the hospital, that I was sick, I'd refuse, the police would pick me up, I'd be admitted to hospital, would still refuse meds, stop eating, go through the review board, get found not capable of making decisions, forced to take medication and start eating again. One time, I was so weak and could not walk so they wheeled my bed down the halls and into the room with The Review Board. The judge and lawyer and the person from the Patients Advocate all came from Toronto so it was a big deal to get it organized and get the right people to come in at the spur of the moment.

One of the meds I was on at first was Haloperidol (Haldol), an older drug which made me sleep all day and night except for about an hour. It made me feel like a zombie. I didn't have much quality of life while on it and after being on it for several years caused mild Tardive Dyskinesia. I ended up with a permanent slightly droopy mouth at times and temporary hand and leg tremors. Another side effect of that medication was weight gain from craving carbs. I went from 140 to 210 pounds while out of hospital only to lose all the weight again while starving myself during my many admissions. In 2013 a study was done which found that out of 15 antipsychotic medications Haldol was most prone to cause extrapyramidal side effects (symptoms that are associated with the extrapyramidal system of the brains cerebral cortex which could include movement dysfunction such as spasms and muscle contractions or Parkinson characteristic symptoms such as rigidity, slowness of movement tremor and tardive dyskinesia, irregular jerky movements). Sometimes the symptoms are permanent. It's not a very safe medication but only takes 30 to 60 minutes to start working.

After they switched my meds, almost all of that went back to normal, being put on a drug called Trifluoperazine (Stelazine) which gave me disturbing vivid, surreal and bizarre dreams. This also complicated my staying on medication while reinforcing my reasons to stay off them. When I was trying not to be medicated, I was putting my fingers down my throat to throw up after taking my meds. Soon after, I was prescribed liquid meds but even then, the nurses were watching me to make sure I wasn't running to the washroom, making myself vomit after taking them. Later, while at my parents' home and later still at the group home, I was manipulating my medication to make it look like I was taking it in case anybody checked. I would take the pills out of the bottle for the day and hide them and when the person checked my pill bottle, they saw that the meds were gone and assumed that I had taken the medication. When the doctor figured this out, I was started on liquid meds even while out of hospital which I began replacing the liquid in the bottle with water. Of course, my well being didn't last long at that point and the doctor, and my parents always knew when I wasn't actually on medication. To me taking medication was like a defeat in that I wasn't being loyal to my religious beliefs. I would later realize that God does not want me to live in fear and taking medication was not contrary to my beliefs. The medication I have now been on for thirty years is called Olanzapine (Zyprexa); on it I don't experience any side effects. It has been a Godsend for me, enabling me to lead a more productive life. Keep in mind that nowadays there are many more very safe and effective medications available. It's staying on meds that many patients have problems with.

In March 1990, after a few months of support and care from family while living at my parents' house and working at the greenhouses I decided I wanted to go back and try living and working in Israel once again. Making all the arrangements I knew a little of what to expect having already been there albeit for a short period of time. Once again, I wanted to work on a Kibbutz, so I applied at the office downtown Tel Aviv after arriving. They advised me "for an older person like you", (which made me laugh as I was only 32 at that time), they would send me to a Kibbutz named Misgav Am in upper Galilee which would take me. Riding on the full bus to my destination I was the only non-army person as there was a base nearby the Kibbutz which was at the top of a mountain range. In 1980, well before I arrived, Misgav Am had been attacked, where five armed militants armed with Ak47's and hand grenades cut the fence between Israel and Lebanon. The militants made their way up the mountain and into the main area of the Kibbutz. Once there, they took hostages. A 2-year-old, and a 38-year-old kibbutz member were murdered. During the attack an Israeli soldier died in a rescue attempt. Four children, a kibbutz member and eleven Israeli soldiers were also injured. Now, there is barb wire all along the perimeter and the ground itself in that area is pressure sensitive as well as other beefed-up security. It would be almost impossible for any intruder to invade now.

Arriving at the Kibbutz, I surveyed the area from a beautiful look-out where you could see the mountains of Syria, Israel and Lebanon. It was gorgeous. There were volunteers from all over the world and I was proud to be one of them. The monthly pay for working was five shekels (two dollars Canadian) a month plus free room and board. A small canteen existed on the property which carried various snacks and foods. My monthly pay would buy a jar of peanut butter or a package of pita bread. Obviously, none of us were doing it for the money but for the experience it offered. One morning I noticed a change in the scenery as all the snow on neighboring mountain tops had melted. One of the Kibbutzniks (the people who live there year-round) explained that spring had arrived, the shift in seasons being very sudden and dramatic. From that day on it was warm, previously being in the 15-degree Celsius range during the day now in the mid 20's, with no jacket required and even warmer at the base of the mountain.

Kibbutz life is rich in camaraderie with volunteers like me having little get togethers in the bomb shelter which sometimes included security drills late at night. Mealtimes in the cafeteria, lunch being the main meal, we'd exchange stories about our lives. Having a set routine with like-minded people was good for my spirit though as I was still in the process of healing and was not feeling completely well mentally but was on medication. One thing that helped my mood was spending weekend evenings dancing in the disco, originally a large chicken coop, located on the property. If no one had told me what it was previously I would have had no idea, it looked much like any other disco with glitz and flashing lights, holding about 300 people with some coming from Kiryat Shmona, a city at the base of the mountain.

I had a variety of jobs while there, including working in the textile industry, as well as looking after and trimming the apple trees. They were a little further down the mountain where we needed an armed escort to drop us off and pick us up. Many times we could hear gunfire and shelling in the distance. Other days I spent working in the textile industry making straps for handbags and packaging little rolls of medical gauze that we had our hands all over. They always had the radio playing. I was tapping my foot away happily when one of the supervisors came by saying, "Stop that tapping it's a sign of contentment! " I laughed at that, and he repeated that joke several times over a few days. This Kibbutz was very self-sufficient having apple orchards in addition to many other food crops, fish ponds, chicken coops, tennis courts, cafeteria, movie theatre and a disco on the property.

An interesting thing about kibbutz lifestyle was that all the kids slept in a hotel kind of environment on their own with some supervision, the parents living in their own houses. I don't know if this was typical for all Kibbutzim but for this particular one that's how it was. Also, on this one, once the boys reached 13 years of age, the girls 12, for their Bar and Bat Mitzvahs had to jump off the cafeteria roof, a two-story building, into a large blanket which was being held by some of the volunteers and locals. This was one coming of age ritual that made me feel uneasy for the mental well-being of these young kids some of them being so frightened that they just couldn't do it but had to keep coming back every day until they made the jump.

I was rooming with a guy from Scotland. One night he told me he had a letter from home and asked me if I wanted to hear it. I thought this was a strange request from a stranger but told him I'd like to hear it thinking it was quite interesting the Scottish expressions themselves and their unique sense of humour. When he saw me taking my medication one night, he asked me what it was. I said I didn't want to talk about it as I was still wary of people and medication, not comfortable talking about it. I never spoke about it to anyone there.

One day, a number of volunteers from England and South Africa were upset with one of the other volunteers in the kitchen saying he had disrespected one of the girls working there. They decided they were going to quit and go to Tiberius and I decided I'd go with them. One of the rules when we signed up at that kibbutz was, we had to hand over our passports for safekeeping to the kibbutz management so that we couldn't just take off thereby leave them stuck. They begrudgingly gave us our passports back, and we headed out to Tiberius. Unfortunately, I stopped eating again and taking my meds. I was not drinking alcohol during this period so when we were in Tiberias sitting outside at a restaurant, I was drinking tea after tea while my friends were drinking-alcohol. I'd had about five or 6 cups of tea when one of my new friends said to me "Hey! Keith! go slow!" (like it was alcohol I was drinking) We all laughed.

After spending the day in Tiberias, we took a bus to Tel Aviv, where I got a backpack hostel room on Dizengoff Street on the main fashion strip. I stayed at the hostel for about 2 weeks still not taking my meds nor eating and hardly sleeping, once again mostly lying in bed all day. One afternoon I went out and bought a felafel sandwich from a street vendor but was too afraid to eat it leaving it by a building with some garbage and a pile of wood in front of it. I noticed a few seconds later a guy who had seen me do this checked to see what that bag contained, I'm sure assuming that there was something nefarious going on being that it was Israel, and my behaviour may have seemed suspicious.

A few days later, one of the girls who worked at the backpack hostel told me that I had to pack up and leave the next day because they had a group coming in and I couldn't stay there anymore. I had a feeling that it was because I was lying around in bed all day, they wanted to get rid of me. I went to another hostel where I stayed for almost a week still not eating or taking my meds. I was experiencing trouble breathing, so I went to a pharmacist and asked for a puffer, surprised they just gave it to me without a prescription. Unfortunately, I was too afraid to use it. Late that evening I walked to the emergency department of the closest hospital and told them about my breathing issue. They came back with a head device to put on me as well as some medication to help me breathe. Again, I was too afraid to use it and refused. They didn't know what to do with me so they just told me I could stay there overnight. As soon as I lay down, I almost immediately fell into a deep sleep.

The next morning, once I'd gone back to the hostel, I decided to take a walk up the street. A young woman backpacker from the hostel followed me, was very concerned and was holding on to me while we were walking saying "What's wrong? tell me what's wrong!" Being overly paranoid, I wouldn't answer her as I didn't trust her and thought she had ulterior motives. She convinced me I needed to return to Toronto. However, before taking her well intentioned advice, I took several cab rides going back and forth to the airport each time not feeling safe and so distraught not knowing what was the right thing to do. So intense was my fear it made me incapable of making a decision. Finally, I got the courage, purchased my ticket and boarded a plane heading back to Toronto via Montreal. Though I was paranoid it was not quite as bad as the first time I had been in Israel.

Once I arrived in Montreal instead of staying on the plane for my connecting flight I got off the plane because of the strong odors coming back. Once again, I was met by security who wondered why I was getting off the connecting flight. I explained to them that I was having a serious mental breakdown; ending up taking a train to Toronto where I got a hotel room for a few days.

Still not eating anything nor properly looking after myself, at one point I was sipping the tap water in my hotel room but even that tasted off and made me throw up. I remembered about The Clarke Institute hospital, walked over to it and tried to get admitted. They had me speak to a psychiatrist. After telling him what I'd been going through for the past several weeks he said I would be fine. They were at a loss as to what to do with me and ended up just giving me a bag lunch and told me I would be fine once I had some nourishment. Of course, I knew I wasn't fine and was reaching out for medical attention. Leaving that hospital I threw the lunch away, called my parents and told them I was coming home, somehow getting to the bus station heading to Thunder Bay. On the bus, I remember noticing a lady in front a few seats ahead of me holding her nose. I'm sure it was because of my odor as I hadn't showered for weeks. I made it as far as Nipigon Ontario, 60 km from home and once again was too paranoid to continue on. All the way from Toronto while on the bus I was looking out the window at the side of the road and things looked very strange and surreal. For hundreds of miles It appeared that there were golden coloured pieces cut out of many of the rock cuts formed strangely and uniformly with round tools. Getting off the bus I took a taxi the rest of the ride to Thunder Bay.

It was early morning when I arrived, and I decided I might be better off checking myself in at the hospital instead of going to my parents' house. There was no one to see me at that early hour so I patiently waited in the reception area. Once admitted I again refused medication and food. They took me before the review board once more and I lost again of course. The lawyer who had been defending me the whole time through all my court appearances was getting impatient with me, and rightly so. At this point I wouldn't listen to her, and really had no defence. I was using stalling tactics so I wouldn't have to take the medication or eat as long as possible while hoping that I would die. My mother had been advocating for me as well writing letters to the hospital administrator and members of parliament questioning the revolving door system of mental illness. She was very frustrated and couldn't understand how I could be allowed out of hospital, when every single time I would go off the medication that would keep me well. She thought there should be a law to permanently force medicate those that are a danger to themselves to keep them well, not wanting me to keep trying to starve myself to death.

Eventually, after once again having been put back on medication I started eating again finally becoming so much better.

There were a lot of suicides of people I knew during my many stays in hospital. One friend's own father who was in and out of hospital himself, committed suicide right in front of him. My friend took his own life a few years later, he himself had just become a father. Another guy tried to hang himself in the bathroom, they had to use the defibrillator on him, and he survived. Staff also warned me about a patient they were concerned might try to harm me. A few days later I was in the shower, and he came into the stall and kicked me in the side taking me by surprise. I was furious and butt naked I ran after him, following him out into the hallway. I tackled him which left us both rolling around on the floor fighting. Since I didn't have much strength from not eating for weeks he had the upper hand. The nurses quickly separated us, one of them received a bad bite mark on his hand from that patient. Unfortunately, that same guy stabbed a woman in a parking lot for no apparent reason a few weeks later. Another patient sliced his own arms up and was walking around the bedroom waving them around as they splattered blood all over the floor and curtains. One day I heard screams coming from the women's washroom shower. I hurried to the nurses station to alert them and they ran in and stopped a male patient from nearly strangling to death a young 16-year-old girl with a bathrobe tie. One young guy used to stand in the middle of the dorm room and for minutes at a time rapidly spin in circles with his arms out. He never seemed to get dizzy. Unlike me with my private, ashamed, rocking in bed this guy was right out there for everyone to see. I think it's possible that his spinning gave him some comfort like rocking to music was for me.

I did make some friends at the hospital. As time went on, we used to pace up and down the halls of the locked ward talking for hours every day to pass the time. I remember on my first admission I was sitting at the end of the hallway of the ward and some of the patients were walking down the hallway towards me getting almost to where I was sitting, would look at me menacingly and turn around and go the other way. They did this several times, but even though I was terrified of my whole situation I somehow trusted that they wouldn't harm me. The nurse sitting next to me said "They seem afraid of you," but I wasn't in any way trying to scare anyone.

TIMELINES I'M NOT SURE OF - 1989 TO 93

I'm not sure at all about the timelines of some of the following paragraphs. The stories happened during my nine admissions then the timeline picks up again after that.

The Nursing staff at the hospital was mostly filled with kind caring people. One evening, a Nurse, Rob, went out of his way to bring in some pickerel fish he had caught and coated with cornflakes. He proceeded to then cook it up in the staff kitchen for a late-night meal for me. For me this was so touching and very much appreciated. Such an act of kindness as I was just starting to eat again.

During one of the times where I was refusing meds and not eating for weeks, another staff member, was working handing out meals to the patients and I decided that I wanted to start eating again finally after weeks of fasting. I took my tray but was still scared to eat, changed my mind and brought it back. I returned a few minutes later after trying to calm my fears and told him that I really did want to eat. He told me to "Fuck off" and get out of there. I felt crushed. Everyone there was well aware that I was literally starving myself to death. I went back to bed and didn't try to eat again for several days. During many admissions when I was not eating, I would go over and over in my head should I eat or should I starve, trying to face the dilemma with courage even though I knew the food tasted like it was poisoned or off tasting and therefore inedible to me. I didn't know which it was or what was going on, my mind still couldn't process things rationally.

Sam and Roch were two of my favorite nursing staff members although there were many that I liked and got along with. Roch was a big burly French Canadian with black hair and Sam also with dark hair was of

Italian descent. Both of them liked to chat with all the patients, were respectful, and I could tell they really cared about the people they were trying to help by being there to listen and talk with us in a caring way. Another staff member was studying nursing while I was a patient and had a way of sitting on a couch by putting both of his legs under him. I don't know why but it struck me as unusual at the time. When I arrived with the police and was escorted to the ward on one of my first admissions he handed me a urinal type canister and said, "This is for your piss" At the time I found it very rude and vulgar, and a hospital admission was already a low point for me without making me feel like I was the lowest of the low. Sometime later, he did warm up to me and was quite friendly.

In another one of my hospital admissions late one night I was laying in bed and someone in the hallway was saying quietly near my dorm room doorway "Get ready I'm coming in, get ready I'm coming in" repeating that over and over then emphasized, "I'm coming in!" as he rushed in, opening my cubicle curtains saying, "At last, I've found you!" The guy in the next bed grabbed him and tossed him out the door. The following day I was warned by the nursing staff who suggested I keep away from him, telling me "that patient thinks you are Jesus," (I had very long hair down to my waist, but I can't remember if I had the beard at this point). That same day I was sitting quietly playing cards with one of the staff and the guy came up to me and said, "You're not him!" (I guess he was thinking that Jesus didn't play cards). A few days later I was walking outside near the property as he came driving by. He was probably only sleeping at the hospital nights and that would explain how he was driving around during the day. Depending upon how well someone was, privileges were granted; like leaving the ward to go to the canteen, going home for a weekend or going off the property until finally getting out for good.

He stepped out of his truck, seemed to come at me in a threatening way, then turned, got back in his truck and left. A few days later he was completely discharged from hospital, and I never saw him again.

There were patients from all walks of life, one telling me that he was a commercial pilot and had hallucinated seeing his wife sitting beside him in the cockpit the last time he had flown. He told me not to tell anybody since his wife actually wasn't there, and he could lose his flying license.

There was another patient that was an accountant, and a Filipino lady whose husband told me she used to sing so beautifully but had become afflicted with Alzheimer's and now was hardly able to communicate at all. Another patient who was always very friendly to me told me he had shot and murdered his wife in the bathtub, saying that so nonchalantly and then laughing about it. It was disturbing to hear. Another fellow, named John, and I would often watch the Toronto blue Jays baseball games together as both of us were huge fans. He was elderly and would get confused, maybe having some form of dementia. One day he was walking around frantically and said to me "Keith I don't know what to do... what do I do? I said, "John, just take it easy, go sit down everything is looked after you don't have to worry about anything." He had a seat and looked relieved to hear he didn't need to worry about things ... until the next time. Luckily, I was able to reassure him. During the four years I was in and out of hospital I met hundreds of patients that were being admitted and discharged over and over again. Most of them like me going off medication.

One psychiatrist (Dr Chakrabarti), would sometimes read to me while I was not well and in bed for weeks on end. At the time I didn't appreciate her efforts but later realized it had been very healing for me. I sent her an email in 2021 to thank her very much for her caring efforts.

Several times I tried to escape from the hospital. One time during the summer I decided I was going to make my break. The ward was usually locked but sometimes the door was left wide open. On this day the door was open, and I nonchalantly snuck out while nobody was looking. I walked down the street to a service station where I called a Taxi, first going to the bank and draining my bank account. I then took the taxi to the town of Nipigon 60 kilometers away getting a motel room for the night. My plan was to rest up, then in the morning I was going to the bus station to leave for Toronto. I was so tired and weak from not eating or sleeping for many days at that point that I didn't have much energy. After I'd been resting at the motel for about an hour I heard a knock on the door, then heard "Provincial Police!" It was the Ontario Provincial Police who had been alerted by the owners that I was hiding out at their hotel. The owner's wife was in the hospital at the same time I was, and he'd recognized me and called them. The police said they couldn't allow me to go to Toronto. Back in Thunder Bay my family had been frantically trying to find out where I was and even called the taxi companies. Much to my displeasure at the time I was taken by the Provincial Police to the Thunder Bay city police and then escorted back into the hospital. Of course, it was everyone looking out for me and the best thing they could have done while having my best interests in mind.

Another day after I was once again involuntary admitted, I tried to make another escape, however this time it was in the middle of winter. Wearing only a light shirt and track pants with running shoes I thought I'd be fine in the cold to hitchhike to Toronto. I ducked underneath the window by the nurse's station, seeing that the door was open for a few minutes. I stepped out into the cold day making my way down the street to a main street. It was about -20 c that day and my ears were freezing. After about 20 min, I couldn't take the cold anymore and returned to the hospital, knocking on the ward door much to the surprise of the nursing staff that hadn't yet noticed I was gone. In later years I thanked several of the staff for looking after me during my admissions and for saving my life.

For most of those hospital admissions I was also afraid of the water which tasted funny to me having a very strong off taste. Mom and Dad would both bring bottled carbonated water for me to drink which for some reason didn't taste nearly as bad though it did seem to have a slight off taste. During my illness my mother always said that she knew when I was off my meds because of a very unique, distinct smell to my body. I noticed this as well and I could always tell when I was off my meds and beginning to go off the rails. I would smell a certain strange smell first on my hands then it would spread to the rest of my body within a few days to a week later. I'm sure this was all related to stress. Another sign that I was becoming ill again, I wouldn't take a shower or brush my teeth as I was so afraid of the water. I was near death several times because to me the food smelled and tasted of a taste unlike anything else so I couldn't eat it. Sometimes it seemed like I was eating something laced with ammonia but 95% of the time it was the other worldly smells and an off taste unlike anything I would smell normally or that I could describe. While not eating for weeks, many hours were spent torturing myself in bed thinking about Mom's very tasty dinners especially the fish and corn on the cob. After several more admissions my psychiatrist asked me what I was going to do after I was released this time. I said, "probably go back to my parents place and work at the greenhouses." His reply was "They don't want you anymore!" I thought it was a very harsh thing for him to say and I'm sure my parents had actually said they didn't want me <u>there</u> living at their home anymore. I was very hurt that my parents seemed like they were giving up on me, but actually they were trying to help me by giving me back my independence. Once released from the hospital it had been arranged that I'd go to a group home. This turned out to be very good for me as I had some social interaction with the people who lived there and visitors. Gayle, a support worker who had been assigned to help me adjust, would take me out for groceries, do banking with me and go out for coffee. She was a lovely kind girl, and I really looked forward to the days that we'd spend together.

1993

There was only one instance of a negative thing happening at the home. One time after coming back from buying some groceries I put my wallet up on a shelf. Later in the day I couldn't find my wallet and was sure I remembered where I'd left it. When I checked the shelf, the wallet was gone. There were random people coming and going while visiting our place so anyone could have taken it. This meant I needed to get all my ID replaced. When the snow started to melt a few months later in the spring, I found my old wallet buried in the snow just outside the front door. The money was missing; however, my ID was intact.

Once again, a few months later I thought I didn't need meds anymore and had stopped taking them for several days. I had also stopped eating, drinking water and showering and shaving. There was some money I was owed that was coming from Toronto, so I thought rather than waiting for the mail I'd go in person and pick it up. It really was just another escape attempt. I left the home without telling anybody where I was going, picked up my money in Toronto and hunkered down in a hotel again convinced that everyone was against and out to get me. (Staying on meds helps me make rational decisions. When I'm off meds my world falls apart).

One day, I went out to walk to a corner store to get some bottled water that I was hoping I'd be able to drink. There were some concrete slabs in front of the store which were moving under my feet, giving me an uneasy feeling inside like it was just another part of a conspiracy. I picked up the water and went back to the hotel, but this water also made me throw up and didn't taste right.

I lay in bed most of the time not sleeping, hallucinating hearing car horns beeping in the distance all day and night long. Eventually, after about three weeks, almost broke again, I gave up, called my parents and told them I was coming home. I returned to the group home still refusing medication and food. Gayle and another support worker came to the home and pleaded with me to go back on medication which I refused. The police were notified so they had no choice but to take me back to hospital. This turned out to be my final admission to hospital. I almost immediately went back on medication and eating and never went back off meds again, finally realizing that I did need the meds and food if I was going to be productive and survive. Staying on medication, being more independant in the group home and with all the love and support from family and a social worker finally sunk in and turned me around over time. It wasn't so much like a light switch turned on as a realization over time that I was loved and cared deeply about. I had regained my will to live, seeing no future in continually being hospitalised.

RELEASE FROM HOSPITAL - 1993

Once released, after my last admission, I wanted to read all the records pertaining to everything that had been decided on about me or had to do with my hospital admissions. My memories about everything in this book came back to me in pieces with help from family, records and just by writing things down and rereading over and over. Supervised by a nurse I had spent a total of five or six hours reading my charts, taking notes and making mental notes. On one of those charts, I noticed that the total number of days I had spent in the hospital was exactly one thousand days over a four-year period. Basically, a little under three years in days spent in the hospital; one hospital stay had been for nine months. After leaving hospital for the final time, I returned as a volunteer, helping patients, giving them a break from the ward by taking them to the canteen or games room, staying with them for conversation. They would relax and seemed to enjoy the company, knowing that I was there without judgment. They also knew I'd been a patient myself and had gotten well enough to leave, giving them hope for themselves. I had keys to the nurse's station and the wards which didn't sit well with the staff until they were certain I was acually well. Totally understandable. It was at the beginning of these wellness years that I started to call Mom every morning to talk about what plans we both would have for the day, what happened the previous day and many other subjects. I still do this every morning to this day.

One day while travelling on the Thunder Bay city bus I passed The Shoreline Hotel and saw a sign out front stating that they had rooms available by the month. I spoke to my worker about wanting to move there by myself. She thought it was a good idea, so I moved in. The hotel had a bar upstairs and a restaurant downstairs and even though I didn't drink it was a good place to hang out and meet people and get back into society somewhat. I remember asking someone who was playing pool in the bar one day what he did for a living, and he proudly said, "drug dealer." It was there that I really started to create a lot of artworks in my room on a table the management had given me for that purpose. Prodding me for a couple months the owner of the hotel kept telling me about how great this new thing called the internet was, and the benefits I would reap by learning how to use it. He persisted for a few months and finally got me interested. Computers further nurtured a lifelong passion for creative design and writing music and without it I wouldn't be writing books.

At one point I had enough artwork to do a show with my canvases. What better place to do it than in the lobby of the hotel. I asked the management if that was ok, and they agreed. One of the owners very kindly built six big 3-tiered wooden easels for me to properly display my artwork making it look so professional. I put together an ad and got a spot in the local newspaper. The show was a huge success and sold eleven pieces. Over a number of years, I was able to do more shows in 3 different galleries in Thunder Bay as well as having a poetry reading in one of them.

During my time living at The Shoreline, I met Mike, (he said 'they' called him 'Mike The Good Guy') a house painter and occasional carnival worker who was also staying at the hotel. Mike and I became fast friends and would often do the bar 'crawl' as he liked to call it in the seedy area of town on Simpson Street. I still was not drinking alcohol but would go for the company and an interesting adventure. One night at a bar called Club 555 two sex workers approached us asking if we needed a 'date' but even though we both declined they stuck around and struck up a conversation. The young woman who was talking to me said she was broke and needed some money, so I gave her the 43 dollars I had in my pocket. She wanted to give me sexual favors in return, but I just told her to keep the money and she didn't have to do anything for me. A few months later while on a city bus I saw her get on with her two young children which made me feel very good about helping her out that night. One day, my Mom had Mike and I over for an afternoon tea. Later, Mike often talked fondly about how my Mom had brought out the fancy little bone china teacups like a real tea party.

When I moved out of the hotel in 1997, I moved into a one-bedroom apartment downtown, continuing to do my artwork in the basement of that house. Slowly I was gaining confidence as a bi-product of creating my artwork. In 1997 in my times of staying steady on the medication my doctor suggested and I agreed that I would try and be weaned off medication to see how I would do. After being on about half the dose of meds for about two weeks I was going backwards and not doing well at all again. This resulted into my writing emails to random people whom I found online that were listed in church directories. Some of the messages were spiritual and religious beliefs, in parts pleading to help starving people. I had good intentions and was hoping more people would step up to help the many homeless people in the world and those struggling with mental illness. A lot of people were open and supportive to what I was writing but there were some people not happy to receive the unsolicited religious material I was sending. I found email addresses for several Hollywood stars and sent to them as well. Only one star replied and said in a short email, "Don't spam me, freak!" Years later (which was quite silly of me) I still had refused to watch his highly popular TV series having resented that limited conversation. I've sort of gotten over it and maybe will someday watch it. Another night I phoned the Vatican after finding the telephone number on long distance 411. First, I called the wrong number. I rechecked the number and tried again. I would guess now that it was the middle of the night as somebody at the Vatican answered the phone. I knew I wouldn't be able to speak to the Pope directly, so I asked for somebody that speaks to the Pope or is close to him. The woman on the phone got quite agitated and shouted, "What do you want?" I said I wanted to ask the pope why with millions of people in the world starving was he living in luxury? Obviously agitated, She said, "The Pope, he knows what he's a doing!" I knew I wasn't going to get anywhere with talking to anybody there, so I ended the call and gave up on that. I also sent a letter to Queen Elizabeth after phoning Buckingham palace to get the address but never heard anything back. Ha ha, I'm thinking that The Royals may get those requests often. I can really laugh at it now but at the time it was all serious. In all my writings and sending things out, one of the people in the U.S.A I had sent to thought I was in distress, which was partially correct, so they phoned the police on me. The Police showed up at my door that night and talked to me for a few minutes realizing that I wasn't really in that bad shape mentally. They said they just wanted to make sure that I wasn't trying to leave the planet. I laughed and I told them no I wasn't.

On one Sunday I went to a church to call them out on religious hypocrisy. It was a lovely service. Before the sermon on the subject of sacrifice the song my "Heart Will Go On" by Celine Dion played which was the first time I had heard it. I was so moved that I cried like a baby with tears streaming down my face. After the service I went downstairs for the social gathering and got into a heated debate with a Dutch fellow. I was arguing about the Roman Catholic Church and said to him "The Pope's not God, you know" Upset with me he replied, "does he think he is?" I was all over the place in my mind and left that church that day not feeling very good about what I had done there.

That month, Dad and I were booked to be going on a trip to the Caribbean, my doctor and I had a discussion and we both decided and agreed that it would be best if I stayed in Thunder Bay. At the time on the lower dose of medication I wasn't stable, shouldn't travel, but didn't need to be hospitalised. My Dad went on the trip with William, one of his brothers, I resumed my normal dosage of medication and got better after about a week or so confirming my need to stay on the original dosage of medication.

Eventually I moved into a three-bedroom house by myself where there was a lot of room for me to write music and create art, which I did almost every day and sometimes into the next morning until the sun came up. I was 40 when my parents bought that house, and it was a time of slowly healing for me. Having a quiet spot to create music and art or sitting in the yard or on the deck helped my confidence grow as I settled in the new neighborhood and gained friends.

In 1999, I took the bus to a bar one night, met a lady and asked her out on a date. When she found out I didn't have a car she ridiculed me saying "You expect me to pick you up?" A few days later I mentioned that story to my mother not thinking anything of it but soon after my parents bought a very nice little used car for me to get around in which helped my self-esteem immensely. Had it not been for the incredible generosity and all the caring from my family I don't think that my recovery would have been so steady or like many others with mental illness maybe not at all.

The Cookhouse Band

In early 2000, I was singing in various Thunder Bay karaoke bars. One night I sang at a Legion bar for the first time. The DJ Jennifer was lovely and had a great voice. I went again the next week, this time her husband Tim was the DJ. Apparently, she had told him that she liked my voice and wanted him to hear me as a possible addition to his band. Tim set up an audition at their home including Lyndy another member of the band. Without Tim and Lyndy hearing me play the drums up to that point I joined "The Cookhouse Band," working together for a few years. This band was the perfect way for me to start working again playing along with such great musicians, Tim on Vocals, Lead, Rhythm Guitar and Banjo, Lyndy on Vocals, Synth Bass and Keyboards and myself on Vocals and Drums. Later, Terry who also had the studio we recorded in, joined the band on Bass. We played jobs in Thunder

Bay and around the surrounding area as well as some of the cottage country areas.

When I first started playing with Tim's band my sister Bev purchased a large van for me to use so I could get my drums around which was a huge help. It was totally unexpected but very much appreciated. Tim and I have a somewhat secret handshake which we kind of discovered by accident. Driving back from a job one night we had just finished our gig in Nipigon Ontario and Tim had said something that we both agreed on. Tim put his hand up to do a high five but in the dark neither of us could see the other's hand clearly. We fumbled around trying to make the high five and that's how it turned into our unique handshake, two hands missing each other four or five times and then our arm going backward. Tim also would say (when something funny happened) "That's in the movie!" joking that we'd be making a movie about the band and our hijinks. To this day conversations on the phone with Tim are filled with much laughter, Tim and I having a similar sense of humour. Elaine and I are in touch regularly with Tim and

Jennifer, getting together in Toronto and Thunder Bay several times since I moved back to Toronto.

One night while playing in Schreiber Ontario, we were just finishing our set and I counted in the original swing rock instrumental we would play each time before taking our break. This time, instead of playing that song Tim broke out into the song Born To Be Wild by Steppenwolf but I was playing the rocky swing beat. Lyndy joined in and the crowded bar went crazy giving us a standing ovation at the end. We finished our set with that but later that night Lyndy was questioning whether what we had done was disrespectful to the original version. To answer that question, a few years after the band broke up Tim was attending The Moondance Jam in Minnesota where Steppenwolf was playing. Tim said he couldn't believe it when Steppenwolf broke into the same jam we did in the middle of Born To Be Wild with 65,000 fans going crazy.

One of the highlights of playing with Tim's band was backing up country music recording star Jerry Palmer for a 2 Night concert. Jerry had a number of hits and I idolized him when I was a kid. Tim's band and I also performed at the Canadian Lakehead exhibition a few times. Our band spent many hours in Terry's (our bass player) studio recording Tim songs. Working on them together as a band were times I'll never forget, and some really nice material came out of those sessions.

One night our band was playing at a club and a young lady came up to me telling me how she was studying social work. So I said, "Oh, so you're going to be a sociopath?" hoping that she would laugh. She said very seriously "Yes, that's right!" I was just kidding around but a half an hour later she walked by giving me dirty looks and wouldn't talk to me anymore. She must have figured it out.

When Terry passed away from autoimmune disease and cancer, we had lost the heart and soul of the band and couldn't imagine the band going on without him. We were devastated. Both Tim and I miss the great writing connection we all had in the studio and how we enjoyed each others playing while we played live as a band.

ANOTHER DREAM

There are about 30 dreams of mine documented with exact dates to the day, having kept paper by my bedside to quickly write them down or jot down song or poem ideas, something I'd done since my 20's. One night in 2001 I dreamt that I was outdoors with a bunch of older people but mostly children. It was a gray and kind of dark sky. I prayed to God to make the sun come out, but nothing happened. Then I noticed a tornado in the distance forming in the clouds. I yelled for everyone to get into the schoolhouse nearby. Once we all got inside, I bolted the door and told everyone to stay away from the windows. A lady who seemed like a teacher pointed to a large mirror and opened it revealing a passageway inside to another planet. We all went through and once we got there; I noticed the sun was indeed shining. My first thought was that we weren't on Earth before but were now. I got down on my knees and twice begged God to hear me and talk with me. Then, I was led to a building where I was shown a paper with names and a grading system where people were judged. I saw some names with 4's beside them and 7's etc. I commented to them that I thought that I was going to go to hell, and they said no, I was not going to hell. There was an 8 beside my name and I was told that I needed at least that to get into heaven.

Another dream in around 2002, I dreamt that I was lying in a bed and a man who looked African was on the other side of the room sitting in what looked to be some kind of Shrine. I asked him who he was, and he said he was The Feather Changer. He floated a large white feather towards me and when I touched it, it changed into a white dove that flew away.

During the years from 2003 to 2006, I traveled to Toronto every spring for a month visiting and trying to get accustomed to being and living in a big city again. During those times I stayed at Global Village Backpackers, a low-priced option which a few years later was sold and converted into a high-end coffee shop. I always stayed in a shared room with 4 beds and was used to that, having shared rooms on the road with bands. Several people I met at the hostel from Canada and over seas I still remain friends with.

MORE HEALING TIME – 2005 TO 2007

Before moving back to Toronto, I was a karaoke DJ at a bar as well as a drum teacher at a music school in Thunder Bay. At the bar I met a lot of really great staff and customers and made several long-term friends. The club had a wide variety of clientele of hardcore devoted karaoke singers. It was always a fun atmosphere, and I would arrive at 9 pm for my 10 pm start to get things set up after finishing my drum teaching job which went from 3:30 to 8:30. My 50 strong drum students aged 4 to 60 included a 12-year-old boy (Michael) with a brain tumour. By using rhythm and isolating exercises for his legs and balance he was able to regain more use of one leg that was affected. This became a great sense of accomplishment for me that in a small way I was able to help him. Around Christmas he came in for his lesson wearing a Santa disguise with moustache, beard and red hat. It was very hot and stuffy in the drum room so halfway through the lesson I asked him if he'd like to take off the Santa disguise and he just nodded his head yes and took it off. It was very cute; I was surprised he kept it on for so long. His grandmother who worked at the greenhouses commented to me during the time I taught him how much his balance and movement had improved and how much he loved the lessons. The world lost a bright light after he passed away several years later when the cancer returned. This news deeply saddened me.

A young 12-year-old blind and mentally challenged girl was one of my favourite students. Although she seemed to really enjoy the lessons, I quickly discovered that she was quite sensitive to certain abrupt sharp sounds like some of the percussion we were using. We worked on a lot of clapping out nursery rhymes and song rhythms and tapping it out on congas or bongos. At one point on one of our first lessons she leaned in and said, "I like you!" which just melted my heart. That made me feel like I was making a difference. Her mother mentioned how happy she was that her daughter was enjoying the lessons.

Eventually I left Thunder Bay in 2007 for good to move back to Toronto. I had planned to teach drums again and possibly karaoke DJ. None of that worked out once I got here because the music schools wanted someone with a music degree and the Djing jobs that were available at that time required having my own equipment. I ended up taking the job of doing background in Film and TV which continued till 2015. It's a very busy industry and I worked up to sixteen long hours a day up to six days a week. There are many people in that business from all walks of life that either supplement a creative lifestyle, to teachers on summer break, to so many retired folks looking to get out of the house, earn a little money and meet new people. Many times, I would come across the same people on set forging bonds and friendships. It was there that I met Elaine in 2007, shortly after arriving in Toronto and we became friends for a couple of years, going out for coffee often. We became a couple in 2009. When the production would wrap for the day Elaine would often fill her car up with people that didn't otherwise have transportation and drop them off at all night bus stops or to the subway. We worked crazy hours and were lots of times in remote areas void of bus routes. We all became great friends over the years. She has been a steady force for me which I never had in a relationship. Before Elaine, I had been in and out of relationships my whole life with the longest one lasting only two years. Elaine said to me at the time, "Two years? what makes you think you could have a longer relationship with me?" She added that her shortest relationship ever was two years and that she's a long term girl. When Dad first met Elaine he said to me "don't blow it!" he liked her so much and knew how good she was for my life.

At this time in my life I was doing artwork and had gotten back to writing music for hours on end, using all the latest technology. I had hired another composer to work with me on two, one-minute instrumentals. He was going through a lot of mental turmoil at the time, and I told Elaine that I saw all the warning signs I had witnessed over the years in hospital and was worried that he wouldn't be long for this world. He was on and off medication, with his Mother continually looking up side effects online and telling him how bad antipsychotic medication was. She spent many hours with him outlining all the side effects that he could possibly get. For someone who is paranoid already that's the worst advice he could have heard, her telling him to stay off medication. He and I had many conversations over the phone and in person with me trying to convince him that the meds would actually help him. I went through this myself going on and off meds so I understood his struggle very well. He was living in fear with or without meds. I was hoping he would survive despite his Mom's negativity and constant interfering but much to my sadness he took his own life. Eventually his mother attempted to sue the hospital that tried to help him. She had phoned me to ask if I would be a witness for her against the hospital, but I told her he needed to be on medication and he took his life because he was not well and afraid of the medication. She didn't want to hear it and couldn't accept that reality.

As a part of my healing and trying to keep busy and improve myself I took six months of photography courses at George Brown College, downtown. This helped my photo work immensely. Over the years I have also been studying music recording and how to properly use Logic Pro recording software on a Mac.

From October 2015 to January 2021, I was blessed to meet another great boss who hired me on the spot at our interview at a local coffee shop. With my background working in various jobs at my families' greenhouses I was hired to look after tropical plants in locations of everything from lawyer's offices, skyscrapers, car dealerships to funeral homes. The funeral homes made me feel a bit uneasy, but other than that it was the perfect job at the time. I've had Colitis bouts over the years, and it eventually got to the point where I couldn't work without worrying about not making it to the washroom in time. The funeral homes were my first stop at around 7 am and there were times I had to run down the hall to barely make it to the washoom. I really loved that job, and it was a perfect fit for me otherwise. My problem was not sticking to the right diet to help myself. For me the foods that trigger a flareup are alcohol, coffee, and any milk products including ice cream. There are a few others like onions and tomatoes that were affecting me, but I do those and coffee now in moderation. Elaine has been great helping me to adhere to a reasonable diet plan. When I first met her, I would often buy two or three chocolate bars and other candy and eat it all at one sitting. As well, I was sometimes having a couple beers a day and eating poorly. I'm still on medication for Colitis but I'm being slowly weaned off it by my Doctor who thinks that by following my restrictive diet I shouldn't have a flareup again. Elaine and I tend to agree with him so we're being very careful now. The times that I have had flareups and been hospitalized for a week were when I was off my diet and doing everything I wasn't supposed to do while being off Colitis medication. My Doctor has pointed me to "The China study" which found in places like Asia they don't have Colitis because they don't do dairy. Right now, I'm managing my Colitis, and everything's been relatively normal to date for me.

I have since signed up to do background again although I haven't taken any days still because of worries about being stuck on the film set and not being able to leave to use the washroom. Out of work for about a year, I was trying very hard to find a job where I could take washroom breaks if need be. I applied at dozens of businesses and did interviews at Canadian Tire, a second hand clothing place, a movie theatre chain and a fast food restauarant where I got a job. After my interview and being hired I stepped out the restaurant door on my way home and my phone tinged. I was stunned to see an email from a professional sports team that I had applied to online a week or so earlier. They wanted to interview me. I got back to her within minutes and told her that I had just accepted a job and wanted to honour that. I thanked her very much for thinking of me, although the sports job was actually the job I wanted in the first place. I did the five hour training at the restaurant and a few days later on my first morning shift they had me cutting tomatoes with a sharp knife and slice pickles in a slicer which kept jamming. It looked like it could take my finger off. I'm a person that cuts himself on forks doing the dishes so when I thought about that and how busy it was while I was garnishing orders and also at times on cash, I lasted only three hours that morning. It was not only those things, I was just so overwhelmed with taking orders. There was so much pressure to get the customers meal just right. It was so fast paced and I was so nervous I squirted mustard all over the side of a burger and onto the wrapper. Now, it was all over my gloves too. By this time, I couldnt even fold the slippery wrapper paper. It remided me of 'I love Lucy' and the chocolate factory episode. I told Garry the manager that I just couldn't do it. Dejected, I left there and went home.

Arriving home, I stuck my head in the door saying "I know you're disaappointed and I am too." Elaine was sitting on the couch facing the door when I came in. I had a brief cry at the door and sat down taking my shoes off. Elaine was so very understanding and supportive and asked "Do you need a hug?" and said "that wasn't the job for you." Once my whole family support group found out about my quitting the job they all, each and every one of them said that they couldn't imagine me working in that enviroment. They just didn't want to discourage me and wanted to honor my decision to take a high pressure job like that. They'd all seen me in a kitchen before. One example was one night while I was helping our son Steve in the kitchen slicing cheese with a very small hatchet like cheese knife it only took about 10 seconds for me to cut myself and need a bandaid. I went back into the living room and left the meal prep to the professionals.

After an hour or so of being back at home, I contacted the sports team again and asked if I could still do the interview. They agreed. My interview the next morning went fairly well but I was a bit nervous and thought that I could have done better. The assistant manager told me that I'd know something by the weekend (in a few days) and said that if I had any questions to email her. About an hour after the interview I emailed her and said that while doing the interview I was a little nervous, had stumbled, and I hoped that she could see some of my strengths. As per Elaine's suggestion I also told them I'd recently (a few days earlier) gotten my Smart Serve certification. Half an hour later I got an email that (much to my disbelief and excitement) I got the job. Since the end of April 2022 I have been working for a Major League sports team in Toronto as a retail sales associate. I absolutely love this job and look forward to every shift and talking to people all day. As well, I often work on cash and find the busy pace exhilarating. Finding the right job is essential to my mental well being and it's true what they say about one door closing and another door opening.

I continue to write music, poetry, do computer graphics and photography, have books on Amazon.com and Amazon.ca and have various products including clothing on Redbubble.com as well as Society6.com.

Something else I've always wanted to do and have been doing now for a couple years with an App called Duo Lingo and another called Lingo Pie is study Spanish. This has been great during the Covid lockdown. Also, for my physical and mental well-being I practice yoga daily. I've done a lot of writing over the years and after publishing a self help book and also a book of poetry, my brother Rob one evening on the phone suggested I write my life story which I thought was a good idea. I started on this book the next day writing out about 30 pages of point form happenings in my life. It turned out to be very therapeutic for me even though the subject matter was difficult at times.

Being a firm believer in manifesting reality,

the more I attempt at doing it the more I'm convinced I'm able to. While I was still living in Thunder Bay prior to coming back to Toronto, I focused on living in a building that had a beautiful overlook of the city. When I first got back to Toronto I lived in a house with a couple of guys. When we first met and were traveling back and forth from movie sets Elaine and I would often pass by an apartment building called the Casablanca, and I'd say the name in a Humphrey Bogart voice. That's the building I ended up getting a one-bedroom apartment in and was just down the street from the house I had shared with 2 other guys. I moved onto the 4th floor where a couple tops of buildings downtown were visible from the balcony. Later on, since Elaine was moving in and we needed more space we moved into the newly renovated top floor that had a huge balcony. It was such a blessing and healing place for me having probably the best all-around cityscape views, especially during holidays with the fireworks exploding all over the city. It was the whole floor to ourselves. We could see as far as Mississauga to the west, the lake to the south, and downtown to the east and south. The north end of the building where our bedrooms were was in amongst nature with a little forest going up the hill providing us with both privacy and being able to look out the bedroom window and watch birds, racoons and squirrel's play. It was a wonderful healing experience and I just loved living there for those years.

Never having my own children, through my relationship with Elaine I have been welcomed with unconditional love and acceptance by her entire family. Elaine's eldest son Steve who is a pilot and cinematographer and his lovely wife Jill who is a teacher have one daughter, Evy, now 13 years old whom was just 9 months when old when I first met her. Her middle son Doctor Michael and wife Courtney and two boys also live in Southern Ontario. Elaine's daughter Laura works in Film and T.V and is also a writer., her partner Sage is a court recorder. All happy and successful in their career choices.

From the beginning I was going to be Opa to Evy, (Grandpa in Dutch) but she was saying Apu instead and that name has always stuck. She asked me one day years later why I was called Apu, like a poo. I told her it was funny she asked as she was the one who named me, and I told her the story how the name came to be. She tried calling me Opa one day but soon after went right back to Apu which I love.

Evy's very creative like her parents and many times we have worked on artwork and other projects together. She asked my opinion about her artwork once and said "Because I'm an artist and you're an artist" which was very sweet. One evening as Elaine and I were over at Jill and Steve's having a visit with Evy, Elaine was putting her down to sleep. I was in the living room and suddenly Evy came stomping back out to me. She adamantly said, "Apu, do you understand what Grammy just said to me? time for sleeping no more talking!" and then went stomp stomp stomp back into the bedroom. Elaine heard the whole thing and hadn't said a word to her about any of that. Evy must've heard that from the caring lady looking after her during the day that her Mom was teaching. The lady had 3 young children she needed to put down for a nap at the same time. We both thought it was pretty funny and still enjoy sharing Evy stories with each other.

Something else Evy tried out on me, one day we were having a conversation and just out of the blue she said to me "Thank you for your sarcasm" ha ha, I laughed at that one, I wasn't being sarcastic at all. We've had many great times. One day when she was younger, she had a balloon that she kept bonking me over the head while I was on my knees and every time I started to move, she bonked me again. We both had huge laughs at that bit of fun. Another time, Elaine snapped a great photo of me on all fours with Evy riding my back like I was a horse with both of us just howling with laughter. It's a wonderful picture which we cherish. These times are so special, especially when she would just out of the blue say to me or Grammy, "I love you." I've often said to Elaine I don't know what I've done to deserve the love of that little girl. She has written beautiful Birthday, Valentine's and Father's day cards to me, making me not only artwork that has a heart and the word Apu in the middle but also a special mug I cherish and a bracelet saying Apu. She has shown me so much unconditional love over the years. I'm honoured to be a part of and welcomed into this amazing family.

LOVE YOU DAD

Watching my Dad go through cancer and losing him to it was very hard for all of us. I thought I knew what grief felt like but when he died, I felt grief like never before. If there is one thing in my life that I regret is that I didn't always take the time to be more inclusive with Dad. Many times, I would call their house, Dad would answer, and I'd only speak to him for a few minutes before asking to talk to Mom. He always had time for us as kids when we were growing up. I did get the chance to tell him I loved him while he was in hospital, but I should have done that way sooner. I made a point since that time to tell my mother, sister, and brothers that I love them.

At Dad's celebration of life, which was attended by over 500 friends and family, I was trying to hold myself together and was doing relatively fine until I saw a good friend of Dads who had been on City Council with him, then I completely lost it and broke down crying. He told me that he didn't mean to make me cry but I think it was at that moment when I saw him that the full gravity hit me. The tribute to Dad was a really heartfelt example of how loved he was by so many people in Thunder Bay. It was such an outpouring of respect and appreciation for the many things that Dad had accomplished in his life including raising a loving family, being instrumental in getting the Community Auditorium built, being on The City Beautification Committee and all his years on The School Board as well as on City Council. Dad was always open to getting telephone calls from anyone who needed assistance. He would listen intently and would do his utmost to do whatever it took to help that person. Hardly a day goes by without me thinking about Dad, and I'm thankful Elaine and her family got to know him, and have the many shared experiences, stories and trips together.

Please Remember

It's important for a person with mental illness to have family love and support and for that family not to give up on them. Your son, daughter, brother, sister or friend with mental Illness has not asked to be unwell. Without my parents fighting for me, and always with unconditional love, I would have starved myself to death. To me, my successes and experiences after age 33 were only made possible by staying on medication, having creative hobbies like painting, photography, and writing music, and the continued support of my family and friends.

At the time of this writing, I've been well for more than 30 years, the same amount of time that I have stayed on my prescribed medication. The medication, a stable home life, regaining hope, having many interests and hobbies, and trusting the support of family and friends is what is keeping me well. It turned my life around... Trust, faith and hope plus one little pill, every day, to give me a life.

EPILOGUE

I'm very thankful that over the years I've had much moral and financial support from family. Without the moral support from them, and my partner Elaine and family I wouldn't now have been in such a good place, spiritually or mentally. Although most families are not in the position to help their loved ones financially to the extent that mine did, just being there to listen or be the voice of reason is equally important. Without a solid family base it's so much easier to fall between the cracks and I'm very grateful that my family kept pushing through believing that I could get better. For more than ten years having a stable home and loving relationship with Elaine I've flourished creativity. This positive situation also has helped immensely with my self confidence knowing that I'm loved unconditionally.

ACKNOWLEDGEMENT

Many thanks to Elaine, Mom, John, Bev, Jill, Karen, Rob and Sharon for your patience with me while reading so many of my improved versions and for all of your invaluable input. Many thanks to my lovely Elaine for helping me with the many rewrites and flow of this book. Thank you Elaine, Rob, Chris and Jeta for helping with editing. Thank you Laura T. for all the links and lending the book on writing, very thoughtfully making many tabs marking important sections. Thank you Leanne for your input and helping jog memories about the Hotel Isabella.

Many thanks to all the spiritual friends that I made on the spiritweb.org chat. Even when spirit web closed many of you have kept in touch with me on Facebook which I'm always thankful and grateful for. My healing times of the late 1990s into the mid 2000s were so much kinder because of your caring and support.
Many thanks to all of you who have come

to my various shows and gigs over the years and to those that have purchased my products, books, artwork, photography and music. Thank you very much Dr. Corcoran for buying two of my paintings during my recovery and for all of your encouragement.

ABOUT THE AUTHOR

Keith Vander Wees

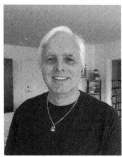

Keith Vander wees has been writing poetry and music since 1977 and creating artwork since 1995. His music is now available on over 200 platforms and 'Funky O' a short instrumental was featured on Dancing With The Stars Australia. Keith's artwork displays have included Toronto's Pearson Airport, a permanent installation in a condo building downtown and a photo in National Geographic 'Dramatic Cloudy Skies.' His work is available at society6.com/keithvanderwees and KeithVander.redbubble.com Keith grew up in the lovely city of Thunder Bay and resides in Toronto with his partner Elaine.

BOOKS BY THIS AUTHOR

A Deeper Hour

Heartfelt and healing prose and romantic poetry with bonus original colourful photos of flowers and cityscapes.

The Immaculate Joy Of Becoming

Self-help and spiritual. Suggestions and ways to improve mental health and overall quality of one's life.

Manufactured by Amazon.ca
Bolton, ON

34006554R00151